MOM'S CANCER

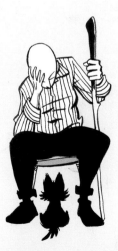

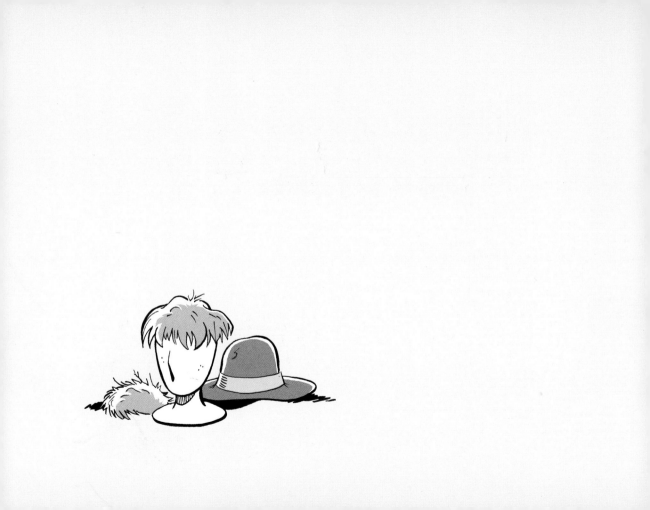

MOM'S CANCER

BRIAN FIES

ABRAMS COMICARTS, NEW YORK

Library of Congress Cataloging-in-Publication Data
Fies, Brian.
Mom's cancer / Brian Fies.
p. cm.
ISBN 978-0-8109-7107-3
1. Graphic novels. I. Title.
PN6727.F483M66 2006
741.5'973—dc22
2005021824

ISBN for this edition: 978-0-8109-7107-3

This edition published in 2008 by Abrams ComicArts, an imprint of Abrams.

Printed and bound in China
10 9 8 7 6 5 4 3

EDITOR
Charles Kochman

EDITORIAL ASSISTANT
Isa Loundon

DIRECTOR, ART & DESIGN
Mark LaRiviere

DESIGNER
Brady McNamara

PRODUCTION MANAGERS
Steve Baker, Stanley Redfern

ABRAMS
THE ART OF BOOKS SINCE 1949

115 West 18th Street
New York, NY 10011
www.abramsbooks.com

To Karen, Robin, and Laura
And Elisabeth, Brenda, and Barbara

Many people have been more supportive of my work on *Mom's Cancer* than necessary, including Jennifer Contino, Otis Frampton, Michael Fry, Joey Manley, Malcolm McGookin, Wiley Miller, Ronnie Pardy, Mike Peterson, Ted Slampyak, Patricia Storms, and Arnold Wagner. Some of them may protest that they did very little; however, even a little at the right place and time can make a big difference. Dad, thanks for surprising me. Special thanks to editor Charlie Kochman.

INTRODUCTION

Mom.

Cancer.

How could the juxtaposition of those two words *not* make us stop and take notice? *Mom's Cancer* is a powerful combination of words and pictures that can unsettle, but in the hands of Brian Fies they inspire.

In a 2001 interview with Stefano Gorla, comics legend Will Eisner said, "I write about what I know and what I have experienced. This keeps me an 'honest' writer."

By the standard that Eisner brought to the field of comics, *Mom's Cancer* is exceedingly honest—and Brian Fies most assuredly writes about what he knows. Not only is his book honest, it is also smart, funny, cathartic, and brave. In the truest sense of the word, it is original.

The world of comics is continuously changing and evolving. Ever since the appearance of Richard F. Outcault's *Hogan's Alley* in 1895, practitioners like Winsor McCay, Harvey Kurtzman, and Alan Moore have been reinventing the medium along the way. The publication of Will Eisner's seminal graphic novel *A Contract with God and Other Tenement Stories* in 1978 paved the road for all others to follow: Art Spiegelman's *Maus: A Survivor's Tale* (1986), Harvey Pekar and Joyce Brabner's *Our Cancer Year* (1994), Howard Cruse's *Stuck*

Rubber Baby (1995), and more recently Marjane Satrapi's *Persepolis: The Story of a Childhood* (2003), have all tested the definition of comics and redefined its subject matter.

Whether *Mom's Cancer* gets added to that list remains to be seen. However, its distinction comes from the fact that it was first created as a Web comic. It was posted anonymously and found its audience online, outside the system of mainstream comics, through word of mouth. A little more than a year later, on July 15, 2005, Scott McCloud presented Brian Fies with an Eisner Award at the San Diego Comic-Con—the first-ever award for Best Digital Comic. *Mom's Cancer* became the Little Web Comic That Could, and it signified a shift in the way comics were made, read, even published.

Although it could have easily continued its existence in cyberspace, passing from one Googled link and forwarded e-mail to another, the story has now coalesced on paper, sold in the traditional arena of book publishing. Our intention is to give *Mom's Cancer* a sense of permanence, and perhaps make it even more accessible, expanding its audience in ways its author/illustrator could never have imagined.

If this is your first graphic novel, we hope you are encouraged to explore the countless others waiting for you to read. Or perhaps you'll be inspired to create your own.

All stories, if they are honest, are universal. Sadly, few things in life are more universal than illness. Each year, approximately 1.5 million people in the United States and Canada are diagnosed with cancer. This is one family's story. In many ways, it is also everyone's story.

Charles Kochman
Editor

PREFACE

You are not alone.

I created *Mom's Cancer* because I wish someone had created it for me. I began serializing *Mom's Cancer* on the Internet in early 2004 as a kind of underground journalism: dispatches from the front lines of a battle into which my family stumbled unprepared. I worked anonymously to protect my privacy and my family, who never asked to become cartoon characters, and also to suggest that the story could be about anybody anywhere. Readership grew by word of mouth. People who needed it found it.

Although *Mom's Cancer* is very specifically about my family and our experience fighting my mother's metastatic lung cancer, I was astonished by how many readers saw their own stories in ours. I was also gratified to get letters from medical professionals and educators saying that *Mom's Cancer* helped them understand their patients' perspectives and asking permission to use it in their curricula. That was an unexpected privilege, as is the opportunity to reach even more readers through print.

When I started writing and drawing *Mom's Cancer*, I didn't know how the story would end. I resolved to be a good reporter and tell it as squarely as I could. *Mom's Cancer* is not a nuts-and-bolts medical manual. Tests and treatments vary; the emotional and practical impacts of a serious illness are nearly universal. Members of my family remember some of these events very differently, and my portrayals of them aren't always flattering. The fact that my mother, father, and sisters still graciously and even enthusiastically support *Mom's Cancer* means everything to me—another unexpected privilege.

    Mom's Cancer is an honest, earnest effort to turn something bad into something good. Although I distrust stories with lessons, here is one: No one will care more about your life than you do, and no one is better qualified to chart its course than you are. You are the expert.

THE CHARACTERS

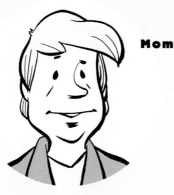

Mom

In her early sixties and diagnosed with lung cancer that metastasized to her brain after a lifetime of cigarette smoking, she is determined to overcome grave odds.

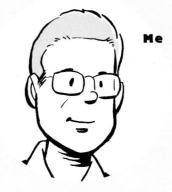

Me

Mom's eldest, a self-employed writer in my early forties with a wife and two teenage daughters, living in the same city as Mom.

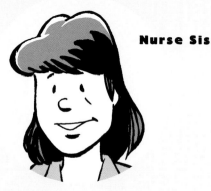

Nurse Sis

One year younger than Me, single, and a registered nurse with years of experience in critical care, intensive care, and emergency room treatment.

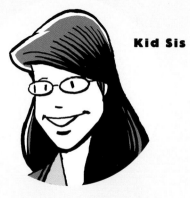

Kid Sis

An actress, writer, videographer, and Web entrepreneur about half a generation younger than Nurse Sis and Me, who shares a condominium with Mom.

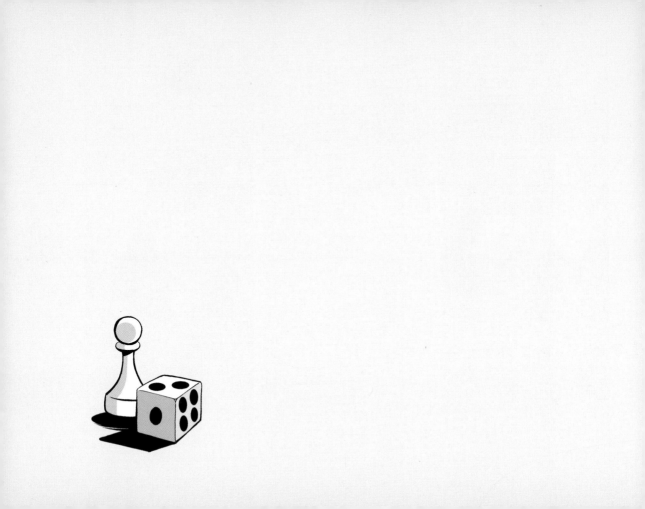

HOW TO DIAGNOSE LUNG CANCER, STEP ONE

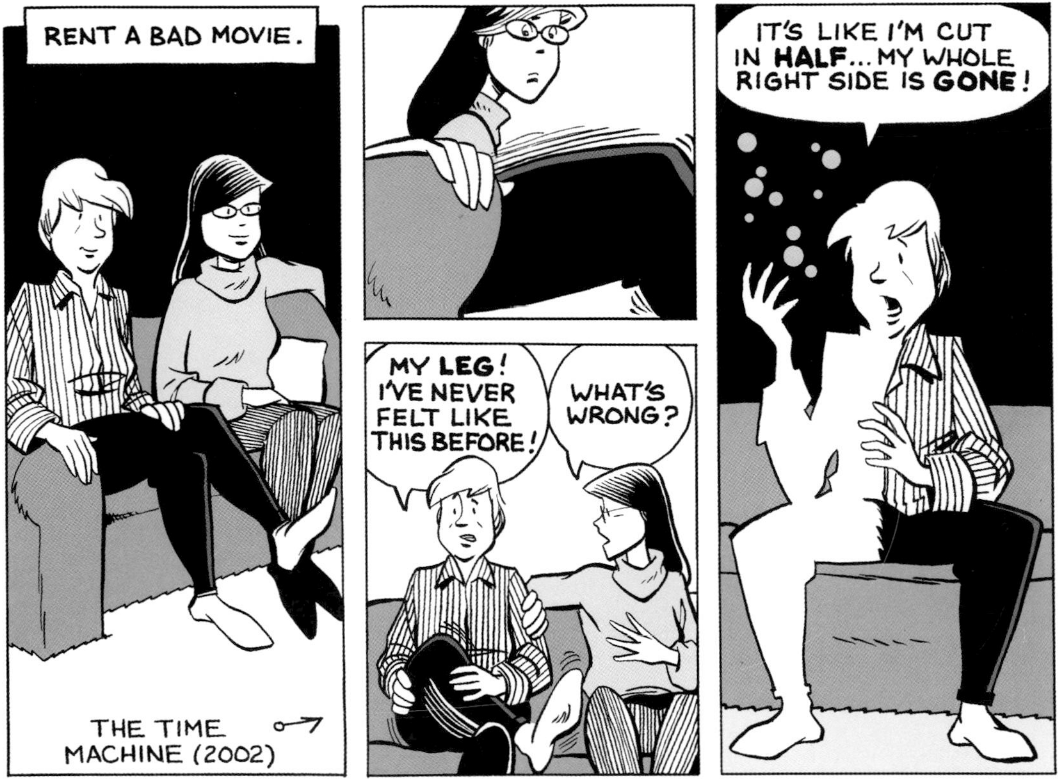
RENT A BAD MOVIE.
THE TIME MACHINE (2002)
MY LEG! I'VE NEVER FELT LIKE THIS BEFORE!
WHAT'S WRONG?
IT'S LIKE I'M CUT IN HALF... MY WHOLE RIGHT SIDE IS GONE!

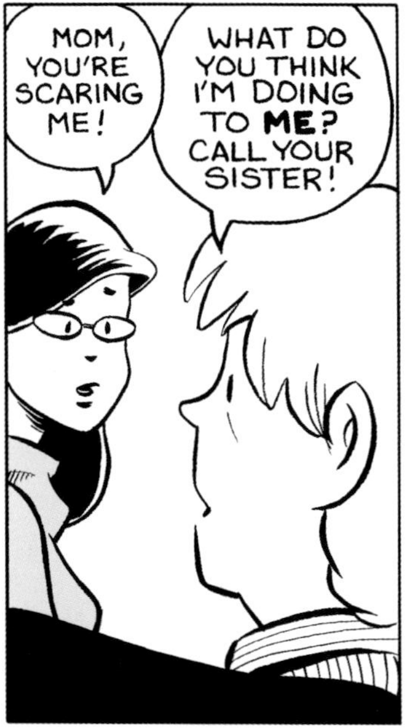
MOM, YOU'RE SCARING ME!
WHAT DO YOU THINK I'M DOING TO **ME**? CALL YOUR SISTER!

KID SIS CALLS NURSE SIS.

NURSE SIS CALLS ME.

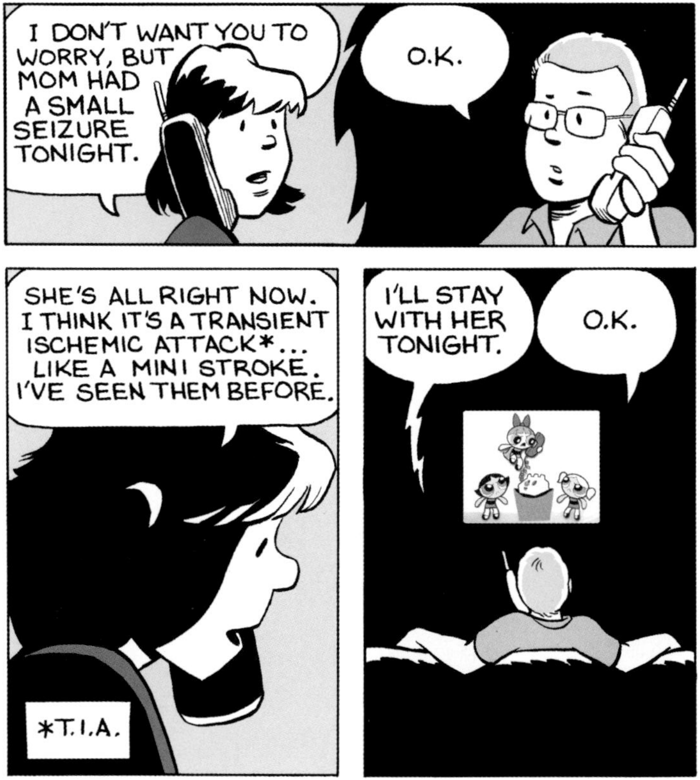
I DON'T WANT YOU TO WORRY, BUT MOM HAD A SMALL SEIZURE TONIGHT.
O.K.
SHE'S ALL RIGHT NOW. I THINK IT'S A TRANSIENT ISCHEMIC ATTACK*... LIKE A MINI STROKE. I'VE SEEN THEM BEFORE.
*T.I.A.
I'LL STAY WITH HER TONIGHT.
O.K.

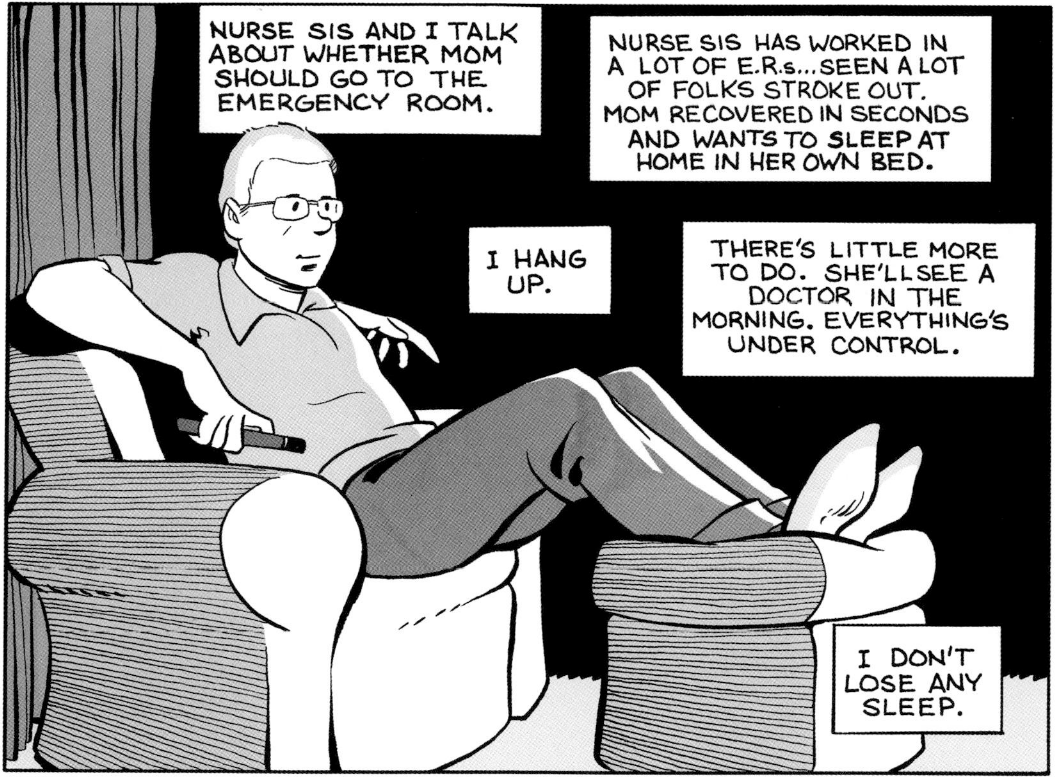
NURSE SIS AND I TALK ABOUT WHETHER MOM SHOULD GO TO THE EMERGENCY ROOM.
NURSE SIS HAS WORKED IN A LOT OF E.R.s...SEEN A LOT OF FOLKS STROKE OUT. MOM RECOVERED IN SECONDS AND WANTS TO SLEEP AT HOME IN HER OWN BED.
I HANG UP.
THERE'S LITTLE MORE TO DO. SHE'LLSEE A DOCTOR IN THE MORNING. EVERYTHING'S UNDER CONTROL.
I DON'T LOSE ANY SLEEP.

HOW TO DIAGNOSE LUNG CANCER, STEP TWO

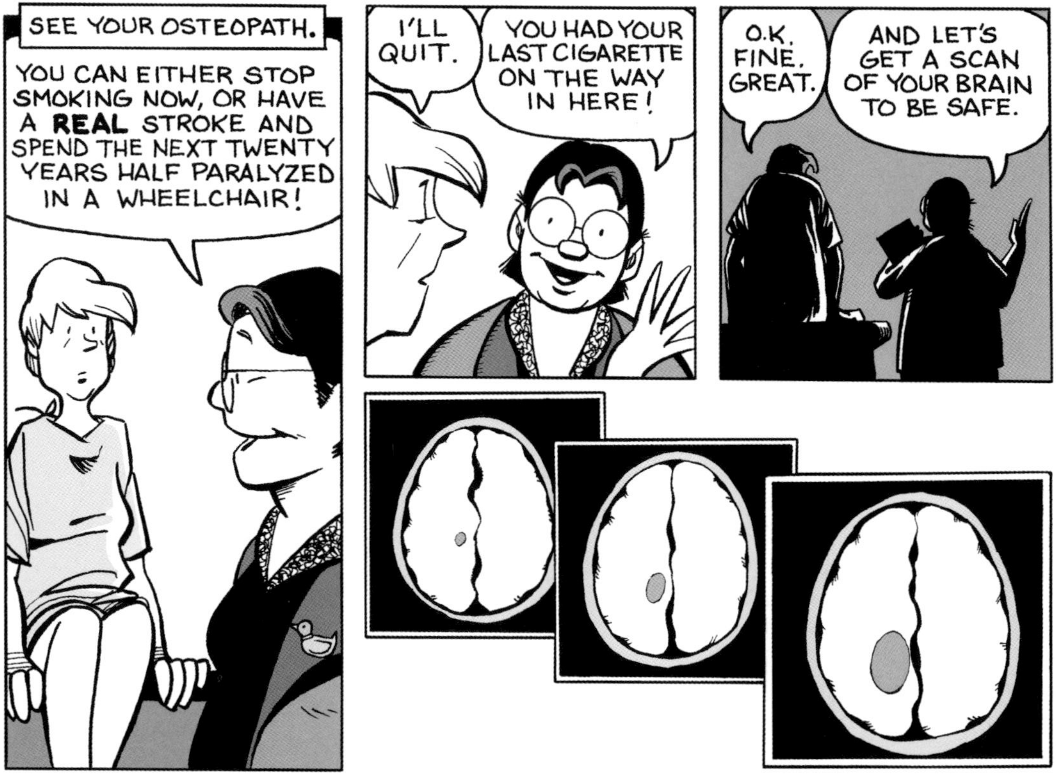
SEE YOUR OSTEOPATH.
YOU CAN EITHER STOP SMOKING NOW, OR HAVE A **REAL** STROKE AND SPEND THE NEXT TWENTY YEARS HALF PARALYZED IN A WHEELCHAIR!
I'LL QUIT.
YOU HAD YOUR LAST CIGARETTE ON THE WAY IN HERE!
O.K. FINE. GREAT.
AND LET'S GET A SCAN OF YOUR BRAIN TO BE SAFE.

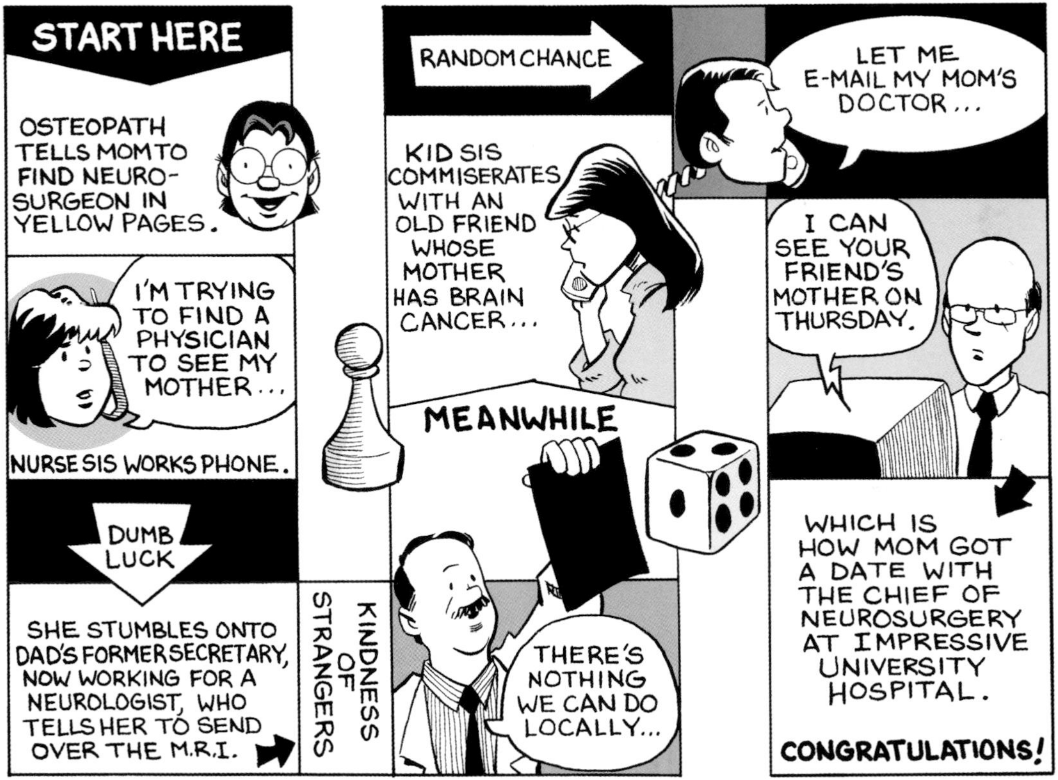
START HERE
OSTEOPATH TELLS MOM TO FIND NEURO-SURGEON IN YELLOW PAGES.
I'M TRYING TO FIND A PHYSICIAN TO SEE MY MOTHER...
NURSE SIS WORKS PHONE.
DUMB LUCK
SHE STUMBLES ONTO DAD'S FORMER SECRETARY, NOW WORKING FOR A NEUROLOGIST, WHO TELLS HER TO SEND OVER THE M.R.I.
KINDNESS OF STRANGERS
MEANWHILE
THERE'S NOTHING WE CAN DO LOCALLY...
RANDOM CHANCE
KID SIS COMMISERATES WITH AN OLD FRIEND WHOSE MOTHER HAS BRAIN CANCER...
LET ME E-MAIL MY MOM'S DOCTOR...
I CAN SEE YOUR FRIEND'S MOTHER ON THURSDAY.
WHICH IS HOW MOM GOT A DATE WITH THE CHIEF OF NEUROSURGERY AT IMPRESSIVE UNIVERSITY HOSPITAL.
CONGRATULATIONS!

LYING IN WAIT

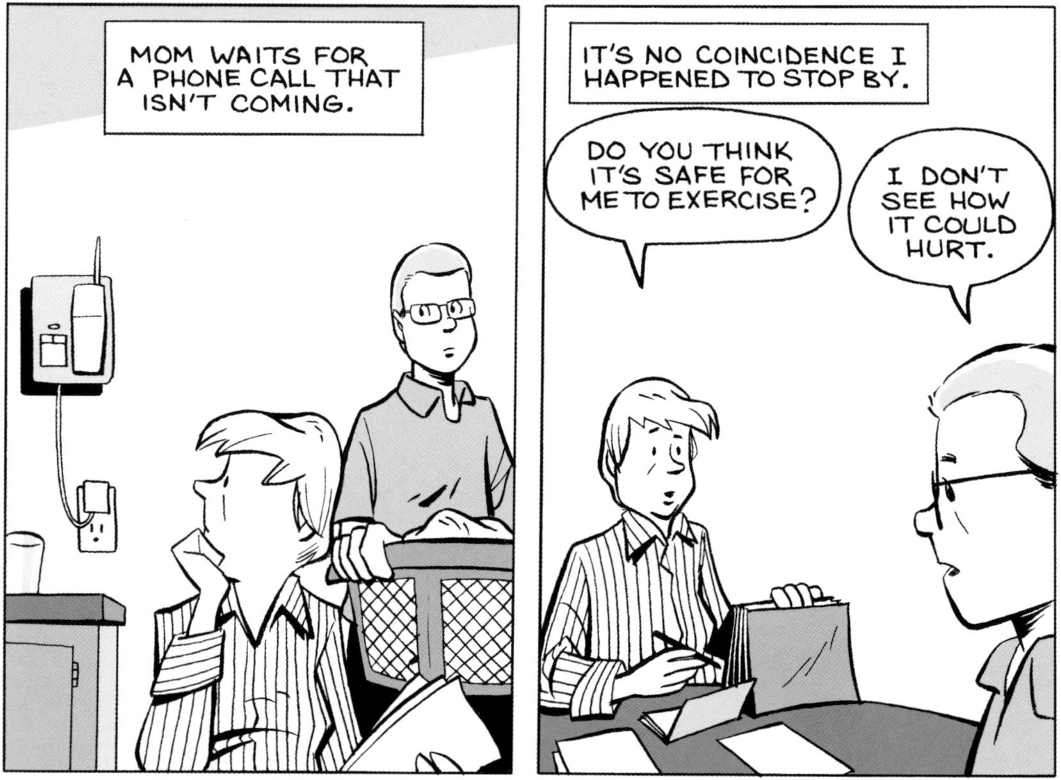
MOM WAITS FOR A PHONE CALL THAT ISN'T COMING.
IT'S NO COINCIDENCE I HAPPENED TO STOP BY.
DO YOU THINK IT'S SAFE FOR ME TO EXERCISE?
I DON'T SEE HOW IT COULD HURT.

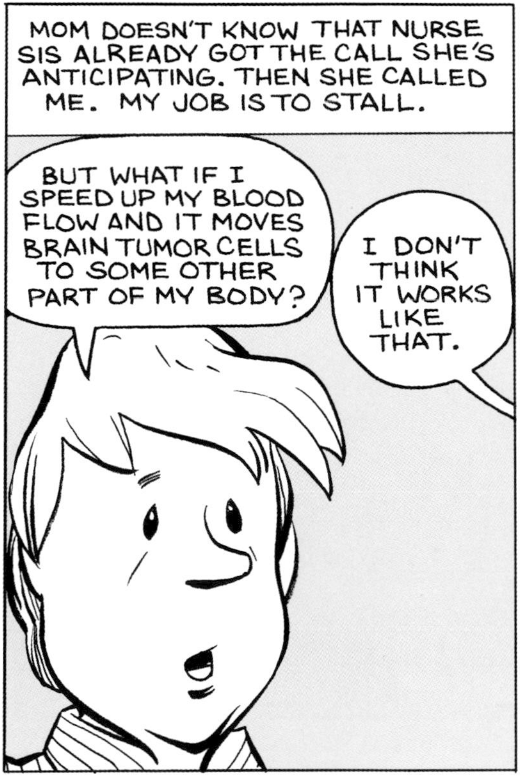
MOM DOESN'T KNOW THAT NURSE SIS ALREADY GOT THE CALL SHE'S ANTICIPATING. THEN SHE CALLED ME. MY JOB IS TO STALL.
BUT WHAT IF I SPEED UP MY BLOOD FLOW AND IT MOVES BRAIN TUMOR CELLS TO SOME OTHER PART OF MY BODY?
I DON'T THINK IT WORKS LIKE THAT.

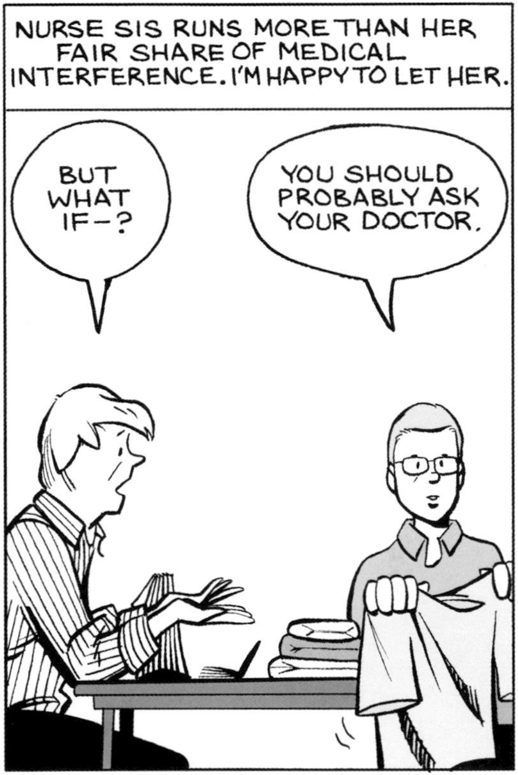
NURSE SIS RUNS MORE THAN HER FAIR SHARE OF MEDICAL INTERFERENCE. I'M HAPPY TO LET HER.
BUT WHAT IF—?
YOU SHOULD PROBABLY ASK YOUR DOCTOR.

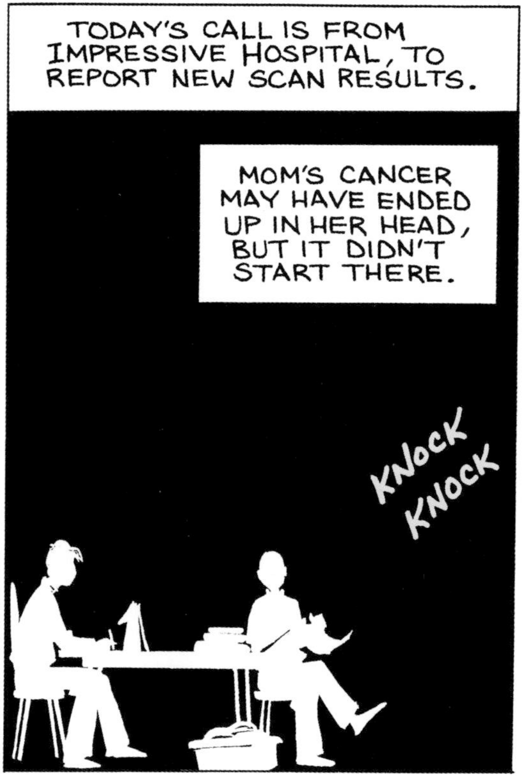
TODAY'S CALL IS FROM IMPRESSIVE HOSPITAL, TO REPORT NEW SCAN RESULTS.
MOM'S CANCER MAY HAVE ENDED UP IN HER HEAD, BUT IT DIDN'T START THERE.
KNOCK KNOCK

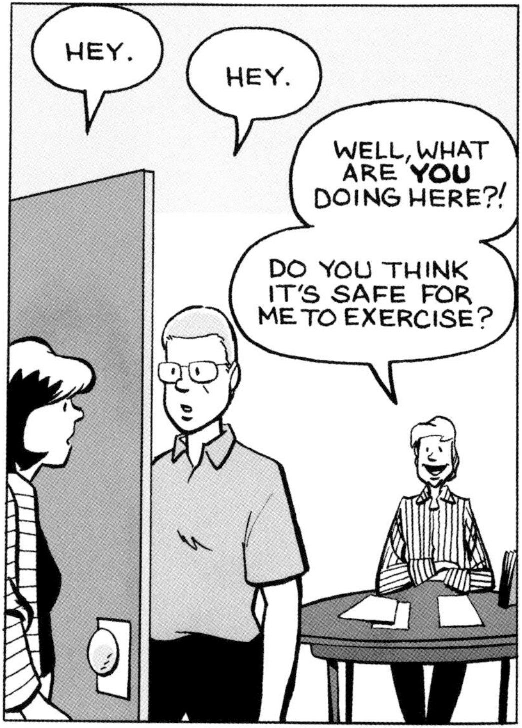
HEY.
HEY.
WELL, WHAT ARE **YOU** DOING HERE?!
DO YOU THINK IT'S SAFE FOR ME TO EXERCISE?

SOME NEWS YOU DELIVER IN PERSON.

A FAMILY MEETING

AMID THE FLOOD OF PHONE CALLS AND APPOINTMENTS, MOM CALLS A FAMILY MEETING.

IT WAS TIME TO DISCUSS SOME THINGS.

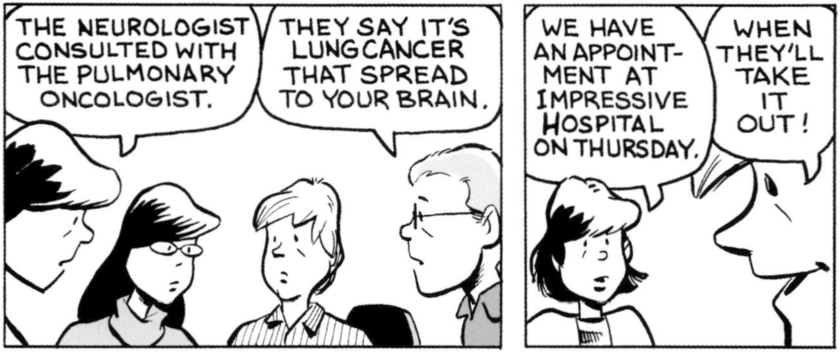
THE NEUROLOGIST CONSULTED WITH THE PULMONARY ONCOLOGIST.
THEY SAY IT'S LUNG CANCER THAT SPREAD TO YOUR BRAIN.
WE HAVE AN APPOINTMENT AT IMPRESSIVE HOSPITAL ON THURSDAY.
WHEN THEY'LL TAKE IT OUT!

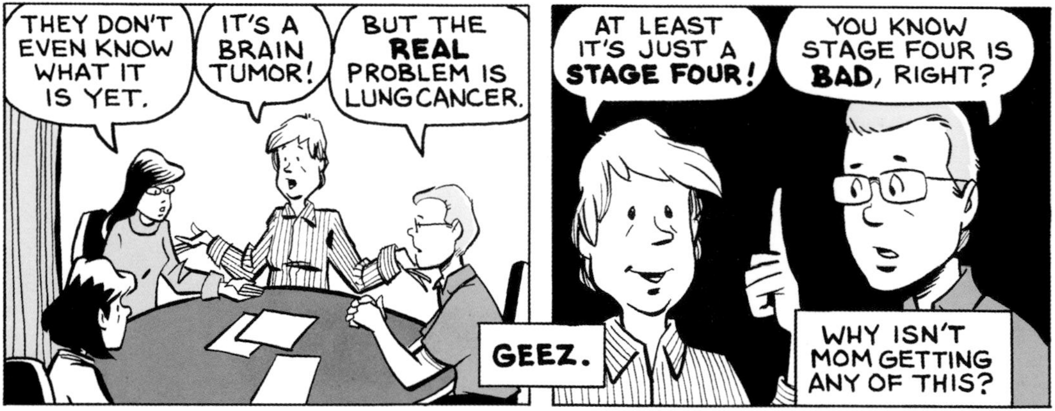
THEY DON'T EVEN KNOW WHAT IT IS YET.
IT'S A BRAIN TUMOR!
BUT THE **REAL** PROBLEM IS LUNG CANCER.
GEEZ.
AT LEAST IT'S JUST A **STAGE FOUR**!
YOU KNOW STAGE FOUR IS **BAD**, RIGHT?
WHY ISN'T MOM GETTING ANY OF THIS?

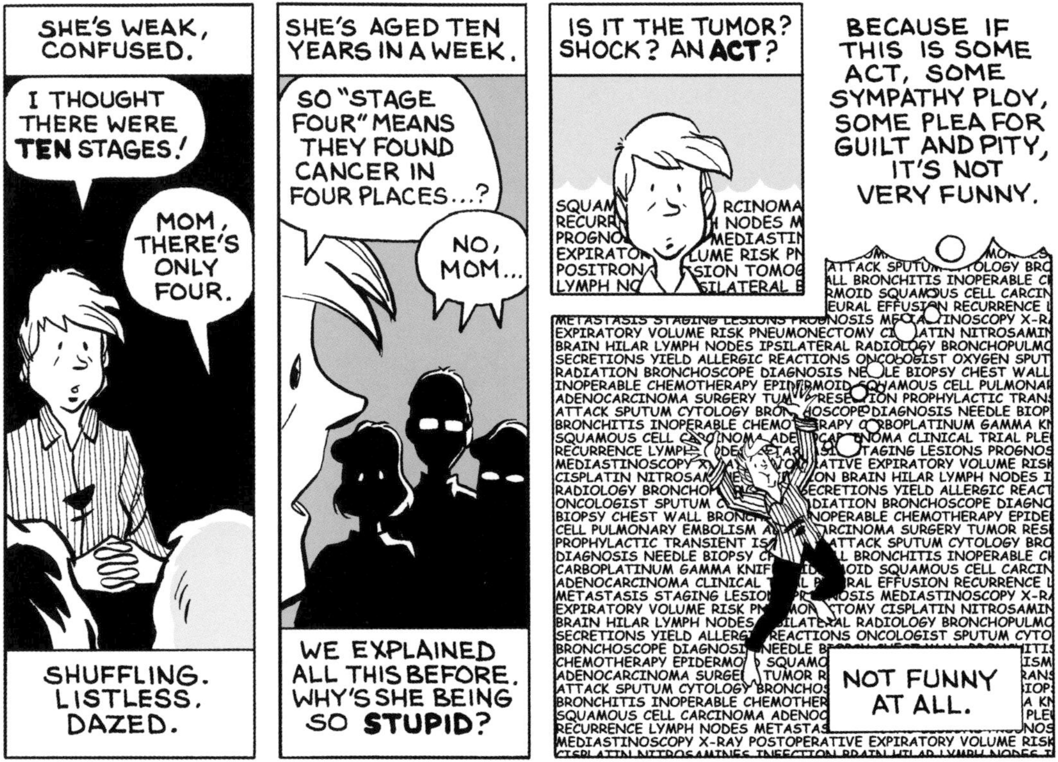
SHE'S WEAK, CONFUSED.
I THOUGHT THERE WERE **TEN** STAGES!
MOM, THERE'S ONLY FOUR.
SHUFFLING. LISTLESS. DAZED.
SHE'S AGED TEN YEARS IN A WEEK.
SO "STAGE FOUR" MEANS THEY FOUND CANCER IN FOUR PLACES...?
NO, MOM...
WE EXPLAINED ALL THIS BEFORE. WHY'S SHE BEING SO **STUPID**?
IS IT THE TUMOR? SHOCK? AN **ACT**?
BECAUSE IF THIS IS SOME ACT, SOME SYMPATHY PLOY, SOME PLEA FOR GUILT AND PITY, IT'S NOT VERY FUNNY.
NOT FUNNY AT ALL.

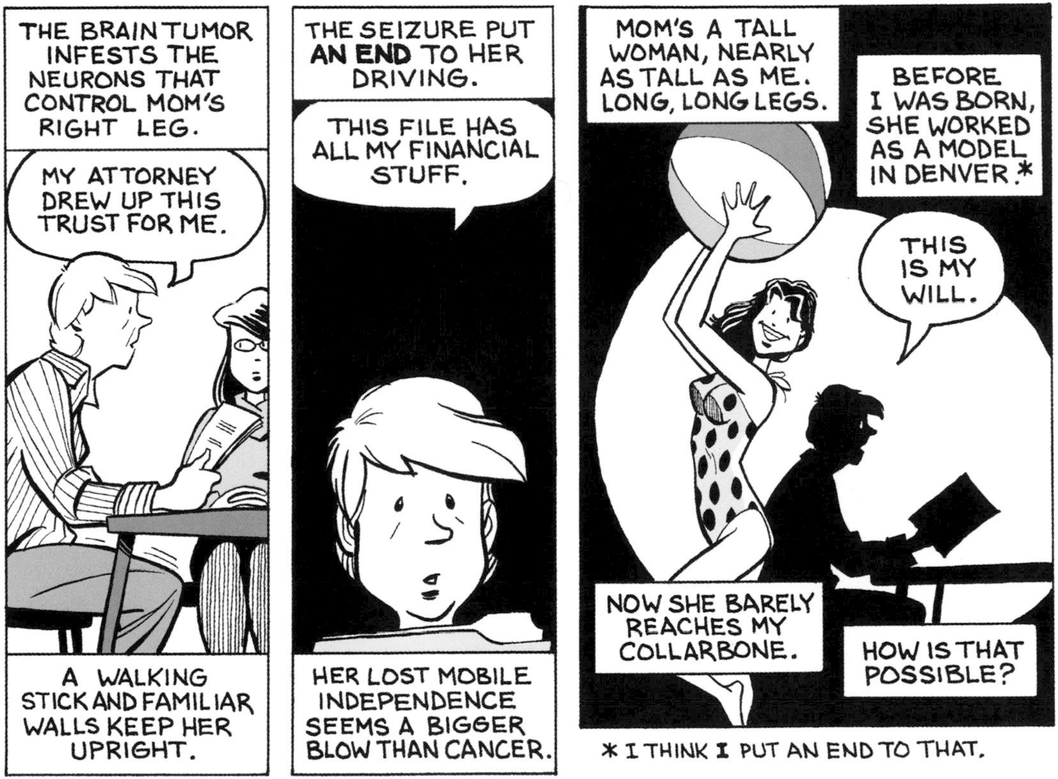
THE BRAIN TUMOR INFESTS THE NEURONS THAT CONTROL MOM'S RIGHT LEG.
MY ATTORNEY DREW UP THIS TRUST FOR ME.
A WALKING STICK AND FAMILIAR WALLS KEEP HER UPRIGHT.
THE SEIZURE PUT **AN END** TO HER DRIVING.
THIS FILE HAS ALL MY FINANCIAL STUFF.
HER LOST MOBILE INDEPENDENCE SEEMS A BIGGER BLOW THAN CANCER.
MOM'S A TALL WOMAN, NEARLY AS TALL AS ME. LONG, LONG LEGS.
BEFORE I WAS BORN, SHE WORKED AS A MODEL IN DENVER.*
THIS IS MY WILL.
NOW SHE BARELY REACHES MY COLLARBONE.
HOW IS THAT POSSIBLE?

* I THINK **I** PUT AN END TO THAT.

INOPERABLE

EVERYTHING FROM MOM'S NECK **UP** BELONGS TO THE IMPRESSIVE HOSPITAL SPECIALISTS.

EVERYTHING FROM HER NECK **DOWN** BELONGS TO A TEAM OF LOCAL CANCER DOCTORS.

BRAIN
TUMOR

SYMPTOMS:

SEIZURE

WEAK EXTREMITIES

FATIGUE

CONFUSION

TREATMENT:

PERIODIC "GAMMA KNIFE" RADIATION

ANTISEIZURE MEDICATION

PATIENCE

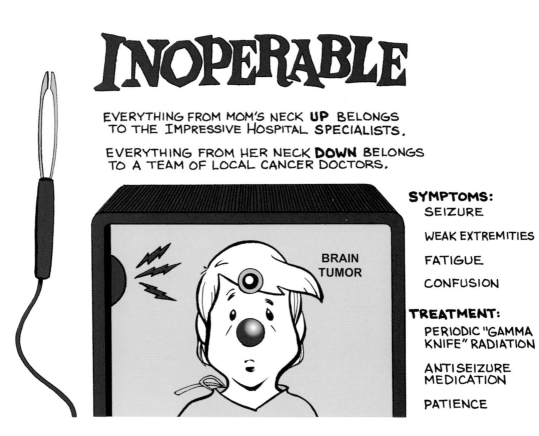

LUNG
CANCER
WATER
ON THE
LUNG

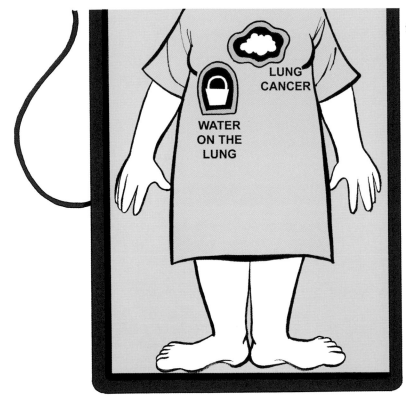

SYMPTOMS:

SHORTNESS OF BREATH

COUGHING

LACK OF STAMINA

FLUID IN LUNGS PREVENTS SLEEP OR COMFORT

TREATMENT:

SIX WEEKS OF INTENSIVE RADIATION WITH CHEMOTHERAPY

FOLLOW UP WITH CHEMO ALONE

DRAIN LUNGS AS NEEDED

REPEAT UNTIL BETTER OR DEAD.

NURSE SIS IS AN AGGRESSIVE ADVOCATE FOR MOM IN THE SAME WAY **SHERMAN** WAS AN AGGRESSIVE ADVOCATE FOR THE UNION.

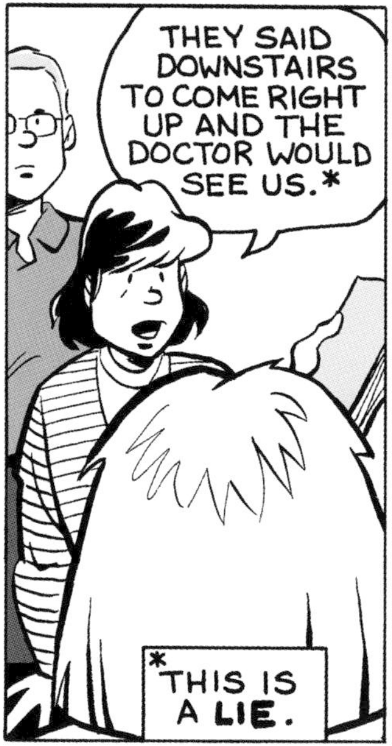
THEY SAID DOWNSTAIRS TO COME RIGHT UP AND THE DOCTOR WOULD SEE US.*
*THIS IS A **LIE**.

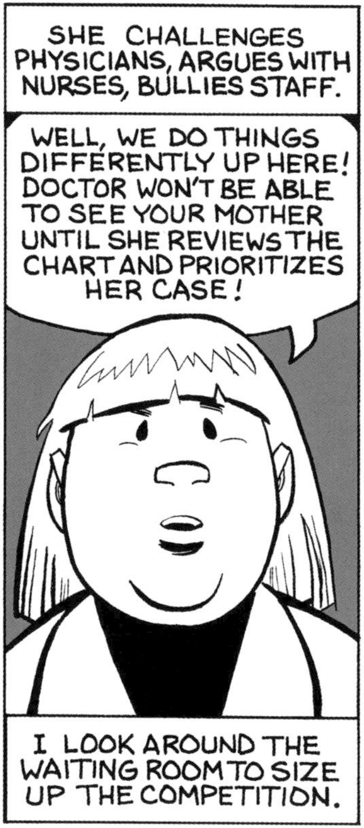
SHE CHALLENGES PHYSICIANS, ARGUES WITH NURSES, BULLIES STAFF.
WELL, WE DO THINGS DIFFERENTLY UP HERE! DOCTOR WON'T BE ABLE TO SEE YOUR MOTHER UNTIL SHE REVIEWS THE CHART AND PRIORITIZES HER CASE!
I LOOK AROUND THE WAITING ROOM TO SIZE UP THE COMPETITION.

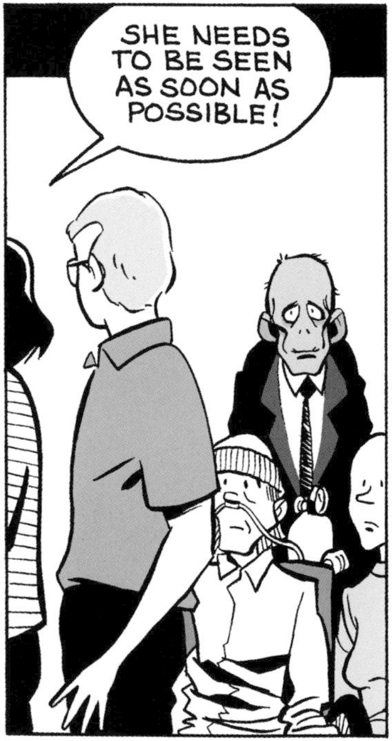
SHE NEEDS TO BE SEEN AS SOON AS POSSIBLE!

NOT AHEAD OF **THESE** POOR SICK SOULS, SHE DOESN'T.

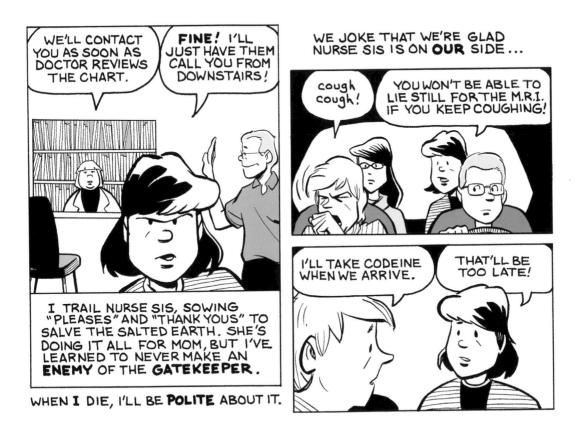

WE'LL CONTACT YOU AS SOON AS DOCTOR REVIEWS THE CHART.

FINE! I'LL JUST HAVE THEM CALL YOU FROM DOWNSTAIRS!

I TRAIL NURSE SIS, SOWING "PLEASES" AND "THANK YOUS" TO SALVE THE SALTED EARTH. SHE'S DOING IT ALL FOR MOM, BUT I'VE LEARNED TO NEVER MAKE AN ENEMY OF THE GATEKEEPER.

WHEN I DIE, I'LL BE POLITE ABOUT IT.

WE JOKE THAT WE'RE GLAD NURSE SIS IS ON OUR SIDE...

cough cough!

YOU WON'T BE ABLE TO LIE STILL FOR THE M.R.I. IF YOU KEEP COUGHING!

I'LL TAKE CODEINE WHEN WE ARRIVE.

THAT'LL BE TOO LATE!

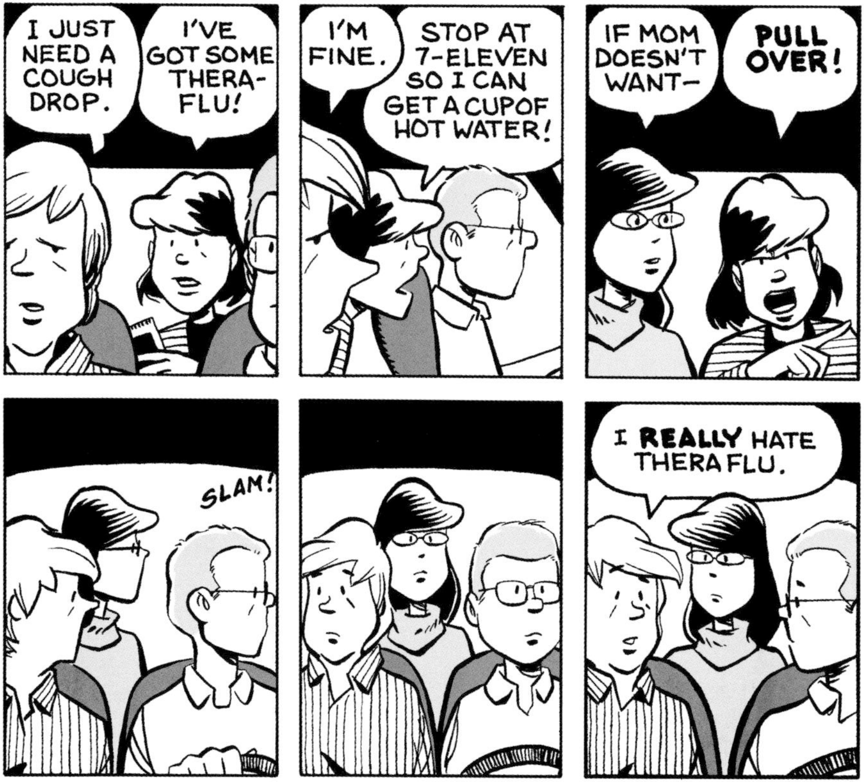
I JUST NEED A COUGH DROP.
I'VE GOT SOME THERA-FLU!
I'M FINE.
STOP AT 7-ELEVEN SO I CAN GET A CUP OF HOT WATER!
IF MOM DOESN'T WANT—
PULL OVER!
SLAM!
I **REALLY** HATE THERAFLU.

DAYS LATER, NURSE SIS SAVES MOM'S KIDNEYS WHEN SHE TAKES OVER AN I.V. FROM A NURSE WHO DOESN'T UNDERSTAND A DOCTOR'S ORDERS.

THE NURSE FLEES THE ROOM IN TEARS ... BUT MOM'S ALL RIGHT.

WE'RE **USUALLY** GLAD NURSE SIS IS ON OUR SIDE.

IMPRESSIVE HOSPITALITY

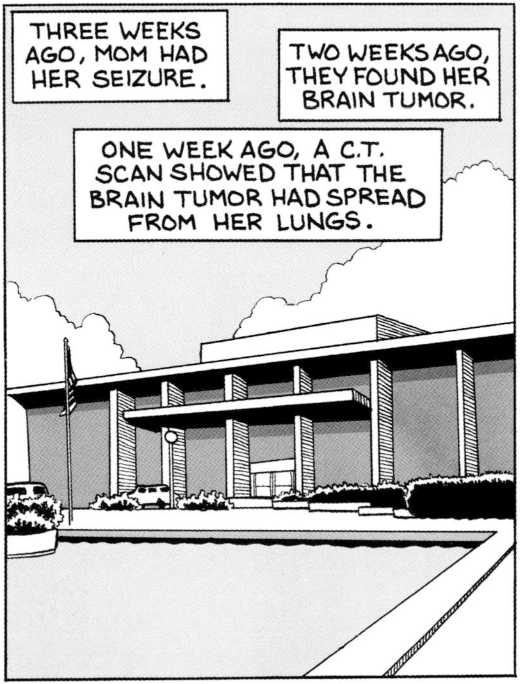
THREE WEEKS AGO, MOM HAD HER SEIZURE.
TWO WEEKS AGO, THEY FOUND HER BRAIN TUMOR.
ONE WEEK AGO, A C.T. SCAN SHOWED THAT THE BRAIN TUMOR HAD SPREAD FROM HER LUNGS.

TODAY WE RETURN TO IMPRESSIVE HOSPITAL TO NAIL DOWN A DIAGNOSIS AND DRAFT A TREATMENT PLAN.

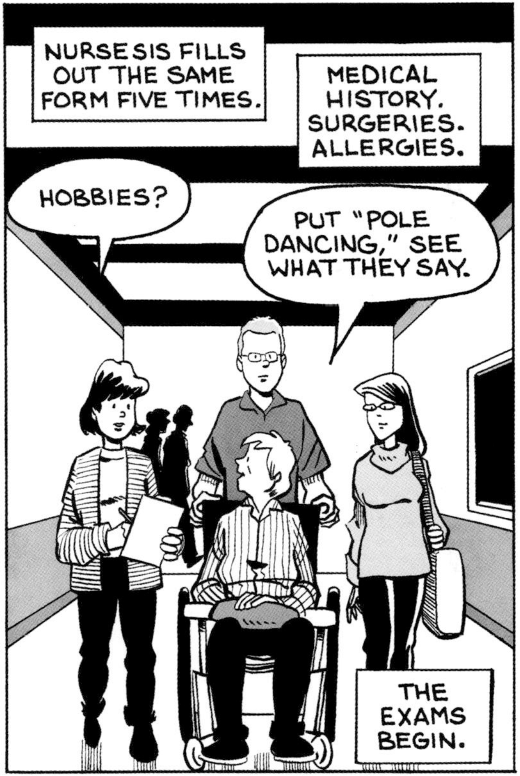
NURSE SIS FILLS OUT THE SAME FORM FIVE TIMES.
MEDICAL HISTORY. SURGERIES. ALLERGIES.
HOBBIES?
PUT "POLE DANCING," SEE WHAT THEY SAY.
THE EXAMS BEGIN.

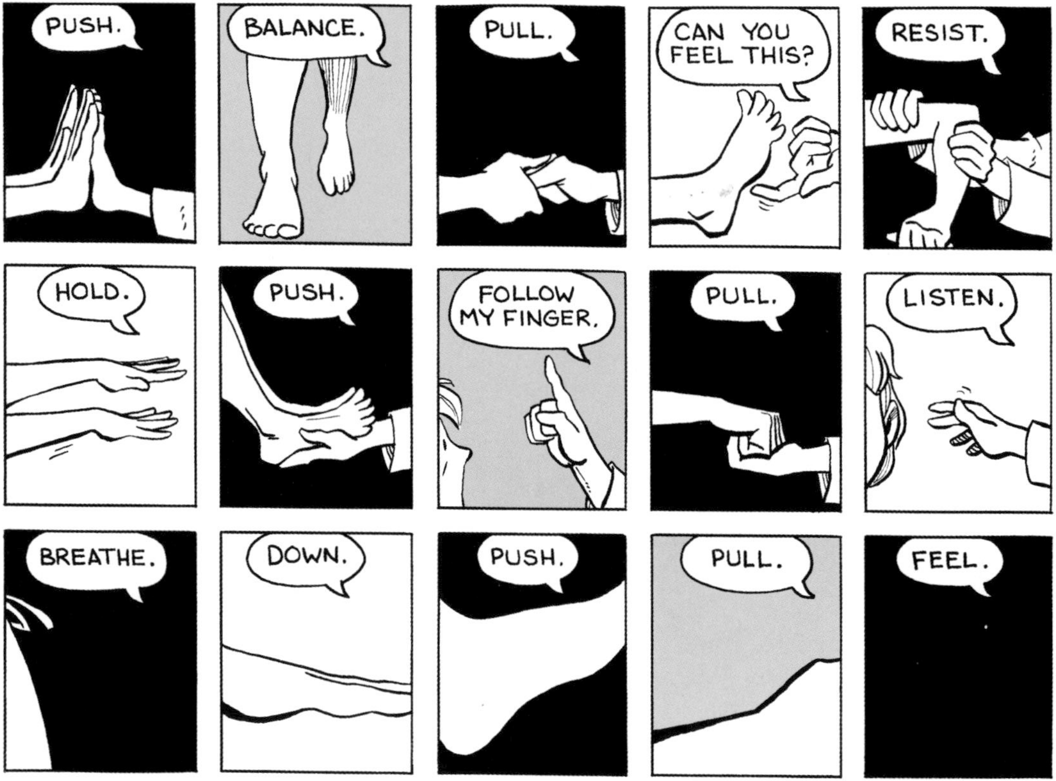
PUSH.
BALANCE.
PULL.
CAN YOU FEEL THIS?
RESIST.
HOLD.
PUSH.
FOLLOW MY FINGER.
PULL.
LISTEN.
BREATHE.
DOWN.
PUSH.
PULL.
FEEL.

18

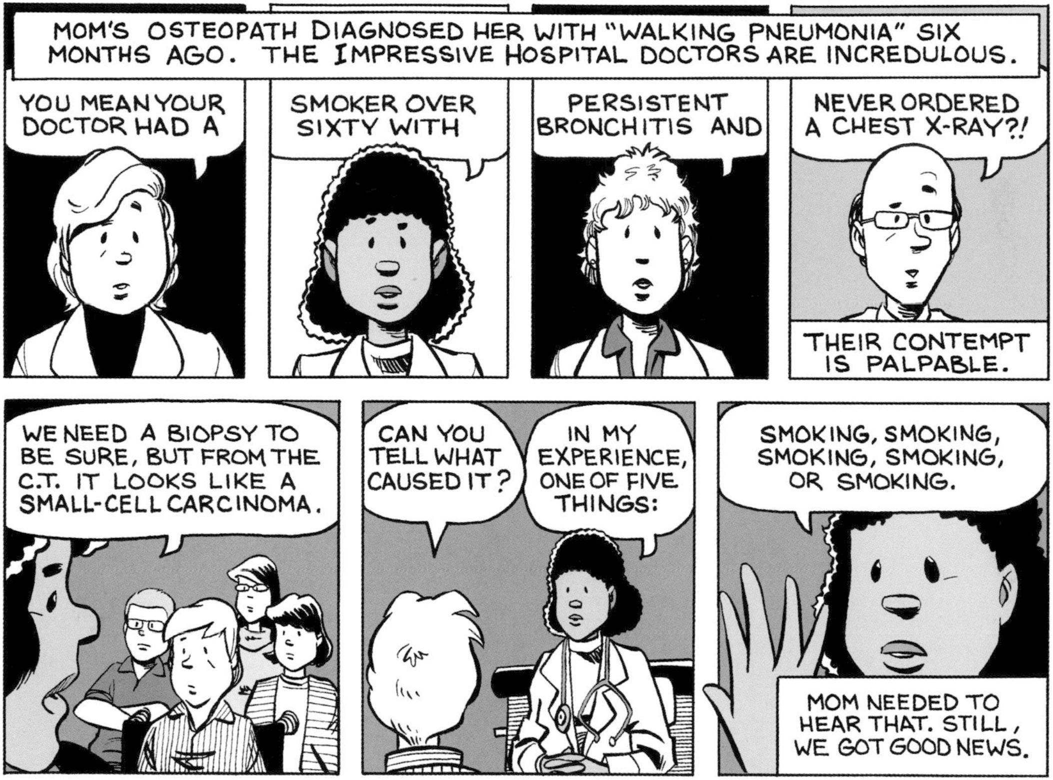
MOM'S OSTEOPATH DIAGNOSED HER WITH "WALKING PNEUMONIA" SIX MONTHS AGO. THE IMPRESSIVE HOSPITAL DOCTORS ARE INCREDULOUS.
YOU MEAN YOUR DOCTOR HAD A
SMOKER OVER SIXTY WITH
PERSISTENT BRONCHITIS AND
NEVER ORDERED A CHEST X-RAY?!
THEIR CONTEMPT IS PALPABLE.
WE NEED A BIOPSY TO BE SURE, BUT FROM THE C.T. IT LOOKS LIKE A SMALL-CELL CARCINOMA.
CAN YOU TELL WHAT CAUSED IT?
IN MY EXPERIENCE, ONE OF FIVE THINGS:
SMOKING, SMOKING, SMOKING, SMOKING, OR SMOKING.
MOM NEEDED TO HEAR THAT. STILL, WE GOT GOOD NEWS.

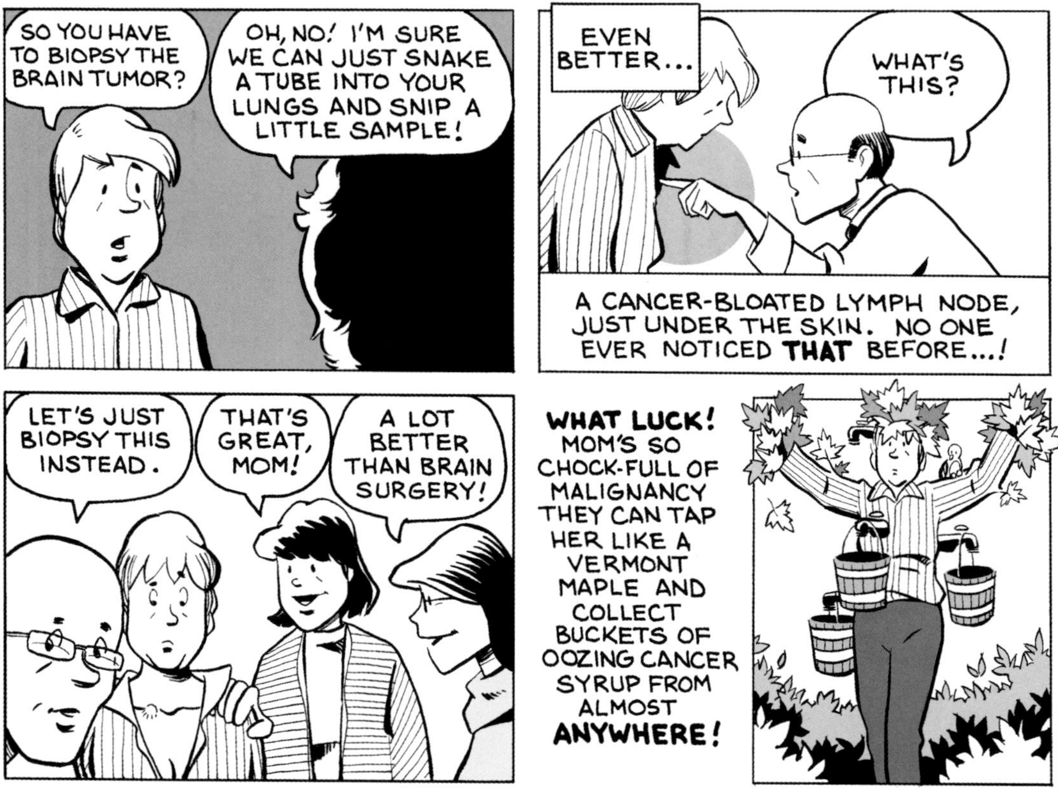
SO YOU HAVE TO BIOPSY THE BRAIN TUMOR?
OH, NO! I'M SURE WE CAN JUST SNAKE A TUBE INTO YOUR LUNGS AND SNIP A LITTLE SAMPLE!
EVEN BETTER...
WHAT'S THIS?
A CANCER-BLOATED LYMPH NODE, JUST UNDER THE SKIN. NO ONE EVER NOTICED **THAT** BEFORE...!
LET'S JUST BIOPSY THIS INSTEAD.
THAT'S GREAT, MOM!
A LOT BETTER THAN BRAIN SURGERY!
WHAT LUCK! MOM'S SO CHOCK-FULL OF MALIGNANCY THEY CAN TAP HER LIKE A VERMONT MAPLE AND COLLECT BUCKETS OF OOZING CANCER SYRUP FROM ALMOST **ANYWHERE!**

DAYS LATER, THE BIOPSY YIELDS A SMALL SURPRISE:

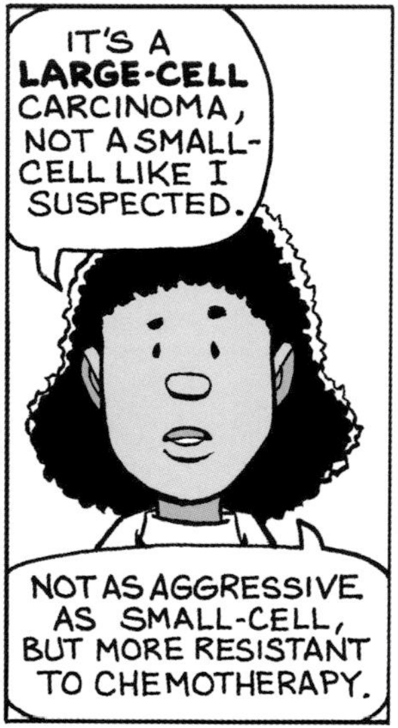
IT'S A **LARGE-CELL** CARCINOMA, NOT A SMALL-CELL LIKE I SUSPECTED.
NOT AS AGGRESSIVE AS SMALL-CELL, BUT MORE RESISTANT TO CHEMOTHERAPY.

IT DOESN'T REALLY CHANGE THE PLAN: RADIATION TO THE BRAIN, WHICH IS IMPERVIOUS TO CHEMO ANYWAY.

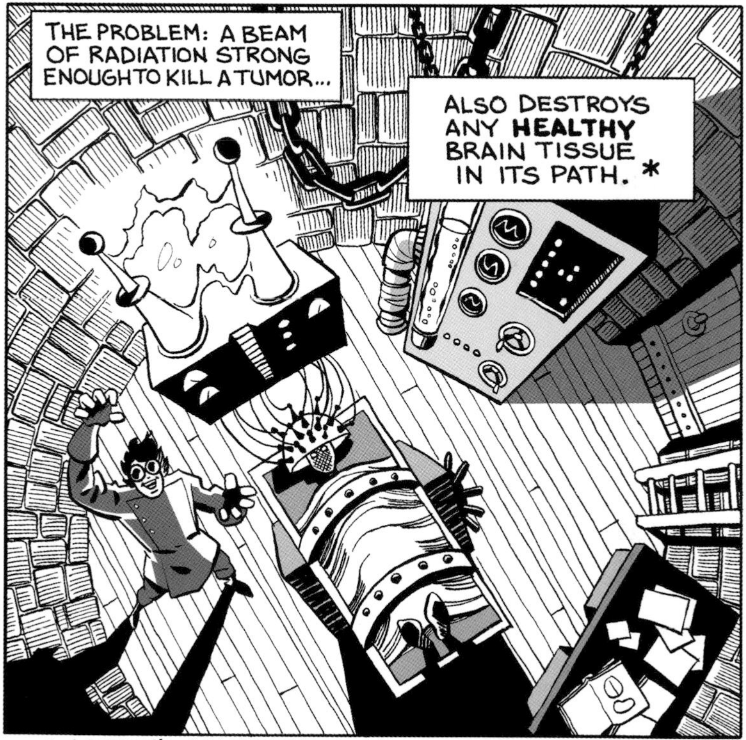
THE PROBLEM: A BEAM OF RADIATION STRONG ENOUGH TO KILL A TUMOR...
ALSO DESTROYS ANY **HEALTHY** BRAIN TISSUE IN ITS PATH. *

* ARTIST'S CONCEPTION. YOUR TERROR MAY VARY.

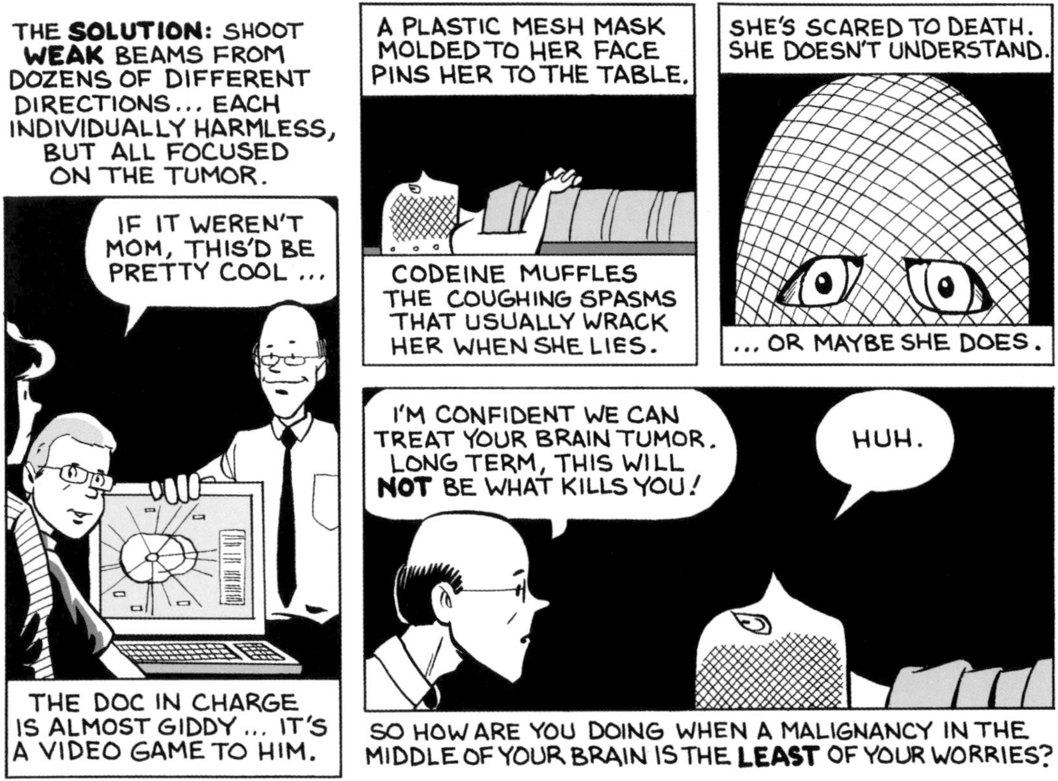
THE SOLUTION: SHOOT WEAK BEAMS FROM DOZENS OF DIFFERENT DIRECTIONS... EACH INDIVIDUALLY HARMLESS, BUT ALL FOCUSED ON THE TUMOR.
IF IT WEREN'T MOM, THIS'D BE PRETTY COOL...
THE DOC IN CHARGE IS ALMOST GIDDY... IT'S A VIDEO GAME TO HIM.
A PLASTIC MESH MASK MOLDED TO HER FACE PINS HER TO THE TABLE.
CODEINE MUFFLES THE COUGHING SPASMS THAT USUALLY WRACK HER WHEN SHE LIES.
SHE'S SCARED TO DEATH. SHE DOESN'T UNDERSTAND.
... OR MAYBE SHE DOES.
I'M CONFIDENT WE CAN TREAT YOUR BRAIN TUMOR. LONG TERM, THIS WILL NOT BE WHAT KILLS YOU!
HUH.
SO HOW ARE YOU DOING WHEN A MALIGNANCY IN THE MIDDLE OF YOUR BRAIN IS THE LEAST OF YOUR WORRIES?

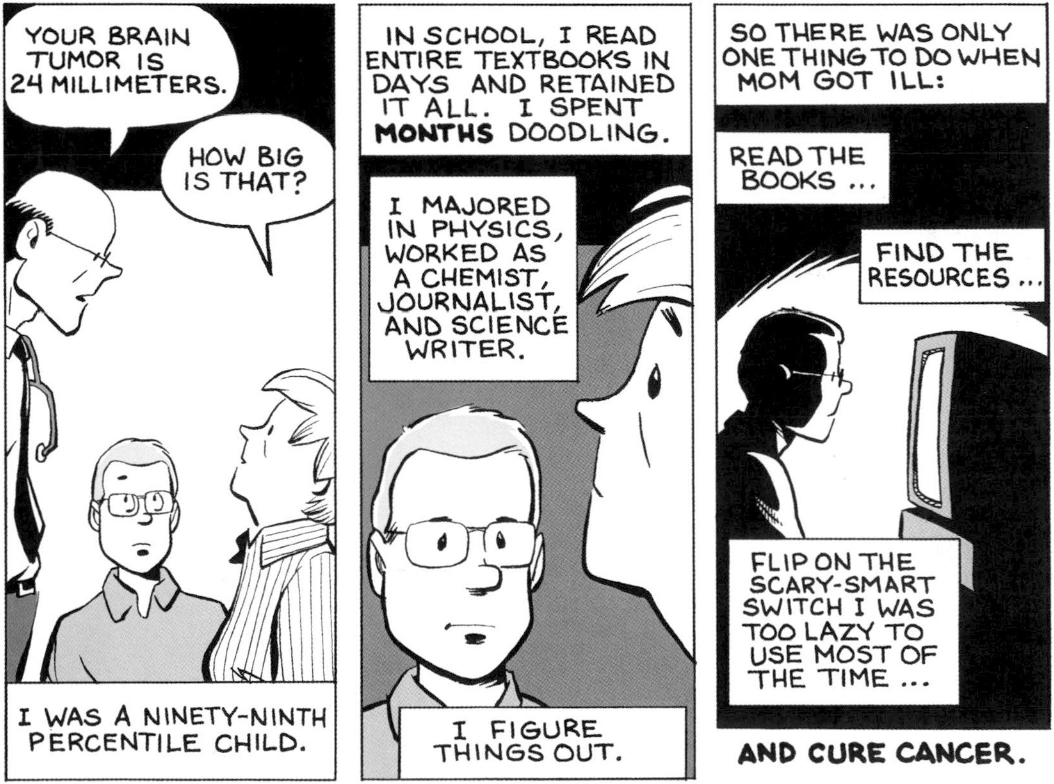
YOUR BRAIN TUMOR IS 24 MILLIMETERS.
HOW BIG IS THAT?
I WAS A NINETY-NINTH PERCENTILE CHILD.
IN SCHOOL, I READ ENTIRE TEXTBOOKS IN DAYS AND RETAINED IT ALL. I SPENT **MONTHS** DOODLING.
I MAJORED IN PHYSICS, WORKED AS A CHEMIST, JOURNALIST, AND SCIENCE WRITER.
I FIGURE THINGS OUT.
SO THERE WAS ONLY ONE THING TO DO WHEN MOM GOT ILL:
READ THE BOOKS ...
FIND THE RESOURCES ...
FLIP ON THE SCARY-SMART SWITCH I WAS TOO LAZY TO USE MOST OF THE TIME ...
AND CURE CANCER.

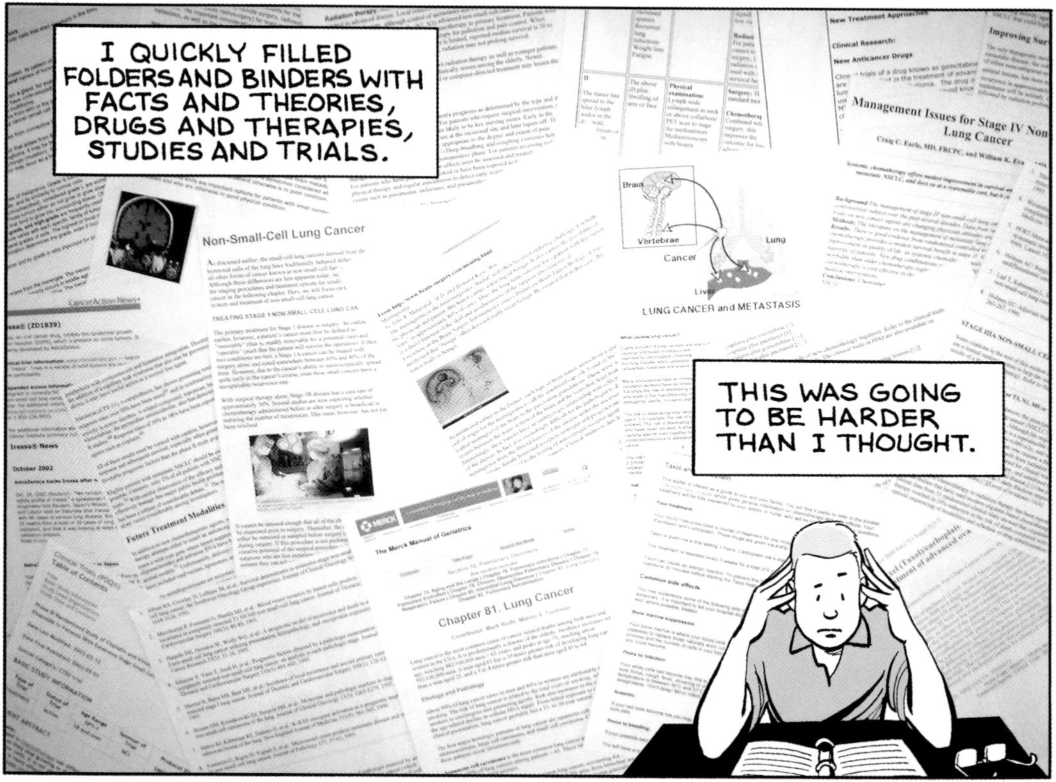
I QUICKLY FILLED FOLDERS AND BINDERS WITH FACTS AND THEORIES, DRUGS AND THERAPIES, STUDIES AND TRIALS.
Non-Small-Cell Lung Cancer
Brain
Vertebrae
Lung
Cancer
Liver
LUNG CANCER and METASTASIS
Management Issues for Stage IV Non Lung Cancer
Chapter 81. Lung Cancer
The Merck Manual of Geriatrics
THIS WAS GOING TO BE HARDER THAN I THOUGHT.

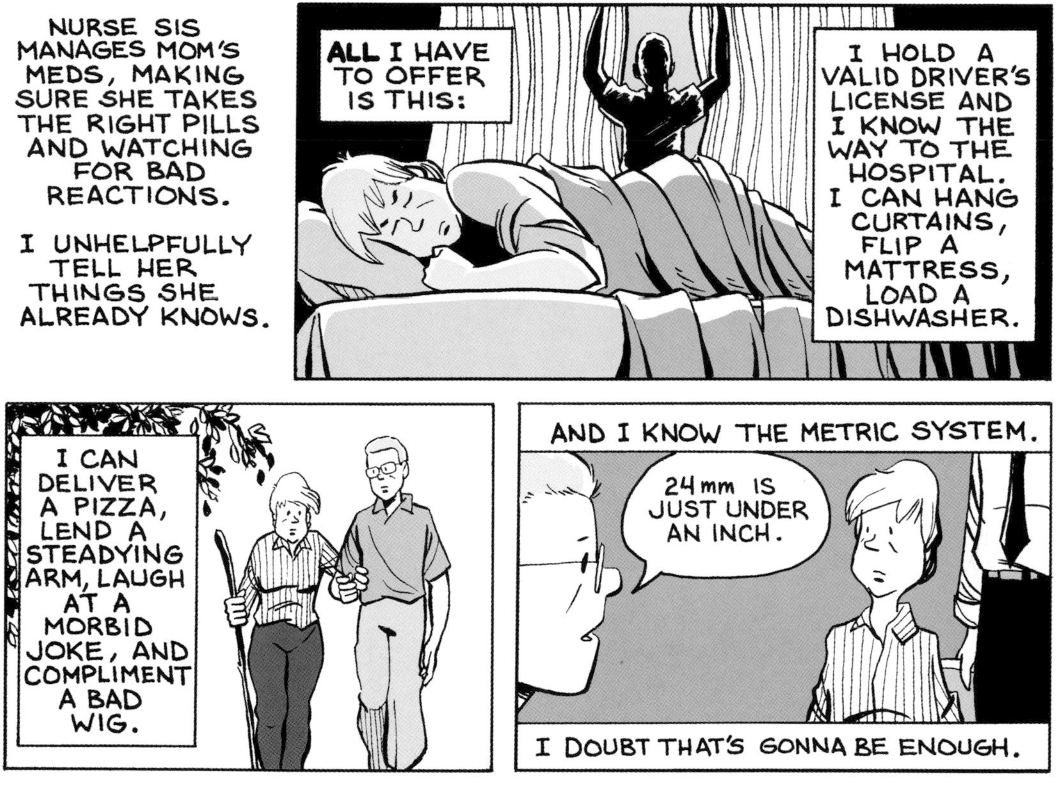
NURSE SIS MANAGES MOM'S MEDS, MAKING SURE SHE TAKES THE RIGHT PILLS AND WATCHING FOR BAD REACTIONS.
I UNHELPFULLY TELL HER THINGS SHE ALREADY KNOWS.
ALL I HAVE TO OFFER IS THIS:
I HOLD A VALID DRIVER'S LICENSE AND I KNOW THE WAY TO THE HOSPITAL. I CAN HANG CURTAINS, FLIP A MATTRESS, LOAD A DISHWASHER.
I CAN DELIVER A PIZZA, LEND A STEADYING ARM, LAUGH AT A MORBID JOKE, AND COMPLIMENT A BAD WIG.
AND I KNOW THE METRIC SYSTEM.
24 mm IS JUST UNDER AN INCH.
I DOUBT THAT'S GONNA BE ENOUGH.

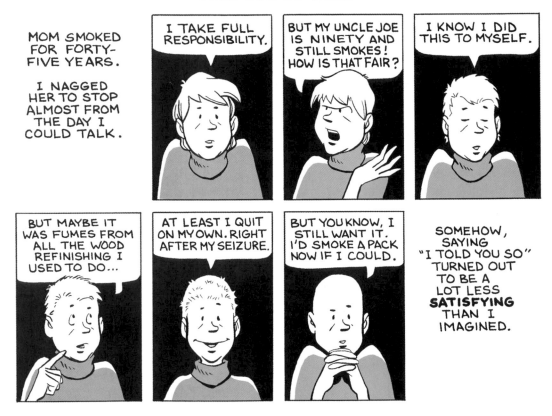

MOM SMOKED FOR FORTY-FIVE YEARS.

I NAGGED HER TO STOP ALMOST FROM THE DAY I COULD TALK.

I TAKE FULL RESPONSIBILITY.

BUT MY UNCLE JOE IS NINETY AND STILL SMOKES! HOW IS THAT FAIR?

I KNOW I DID THIS TO MYSELF.

BUT MAYBE IT WAS FUMES FROM ALL THE WOOD REFINISHING I USED TO DO...

AT LEAST I QUIT ON MY OWN. RIGHT AFTER MY SEIZURE.

BUT YOU KNOW, I STILL WANT IT. I'D SMOKE A PACK NOW IF I COULD.

SOMEHOW, SAYING "I TOLD YOU SO" TURNED OUT TO BE A LOT LESS **SATISFYING** THAN I IMAGINED.

26

KID SIS AND HOLLYWOOD

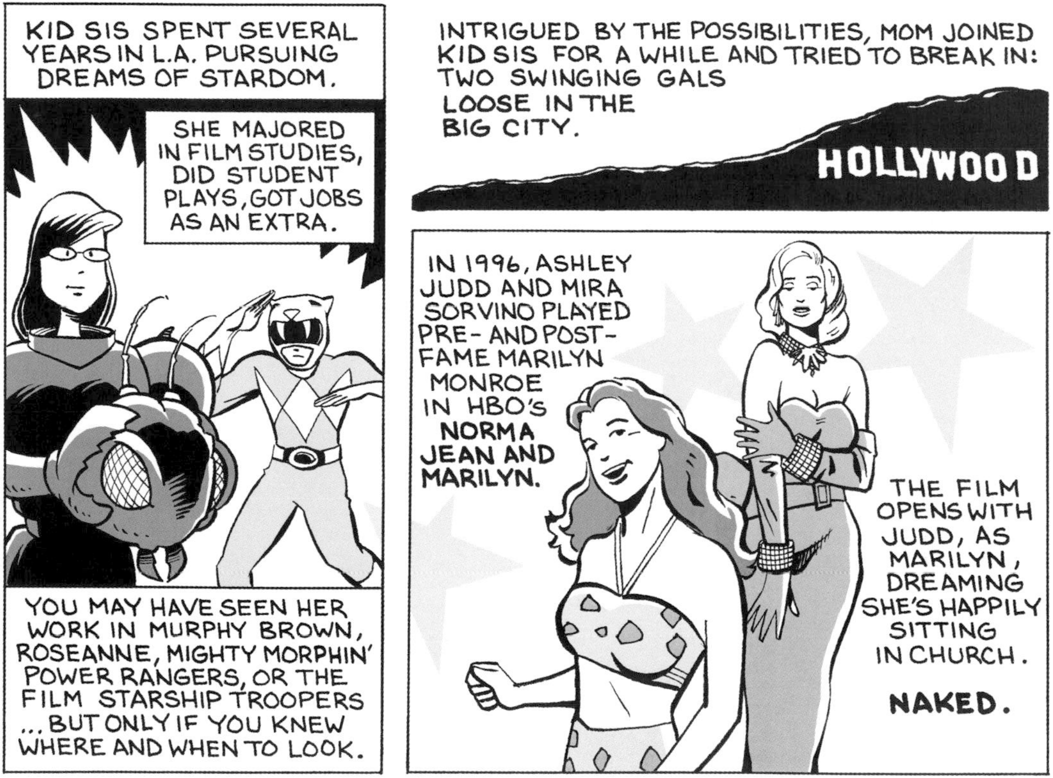
KID SIS SPENT SEVERAL YEARS IN L.A. PURSUING DREAMS OF STARDOM.
SHE MAJORED IN FILM STUDIES, DID STUDENT PLAYS, GOT JOBS AS AN EXTRA.
YOU MAY HAVE SEEN HER WORK IN MURPHY BROWN, ROSEANNE, MIGHTY MORPHIN' POWER RANGERS, OR THE FILM STARSHIP TROOPERS ...BUT ONLY IF YOU KNEW WHERE AND WHEN TO LOOK.
INTRIGUED BY THE POSSIBILITIES, MOM JOINED KID SIS FOR A WHILE AND TRIED TO BREAK IN: TWO SWINGING GALS LOOSE IN THE BIG CITY.
HOLLYWOOD
IN 1996, ASHLEY JUDD AND MIRA SORVINO PLAYED PRE- AND POST-FAME MARILYN MONROE IN HBO'S **NORMA JEAN AND MARILYN.**
THE FILM OPENS WITH JUDD, AS MARILYN, DREAMING SHE'S HAPPILY SITTING IN CHURCH.
NAKED.

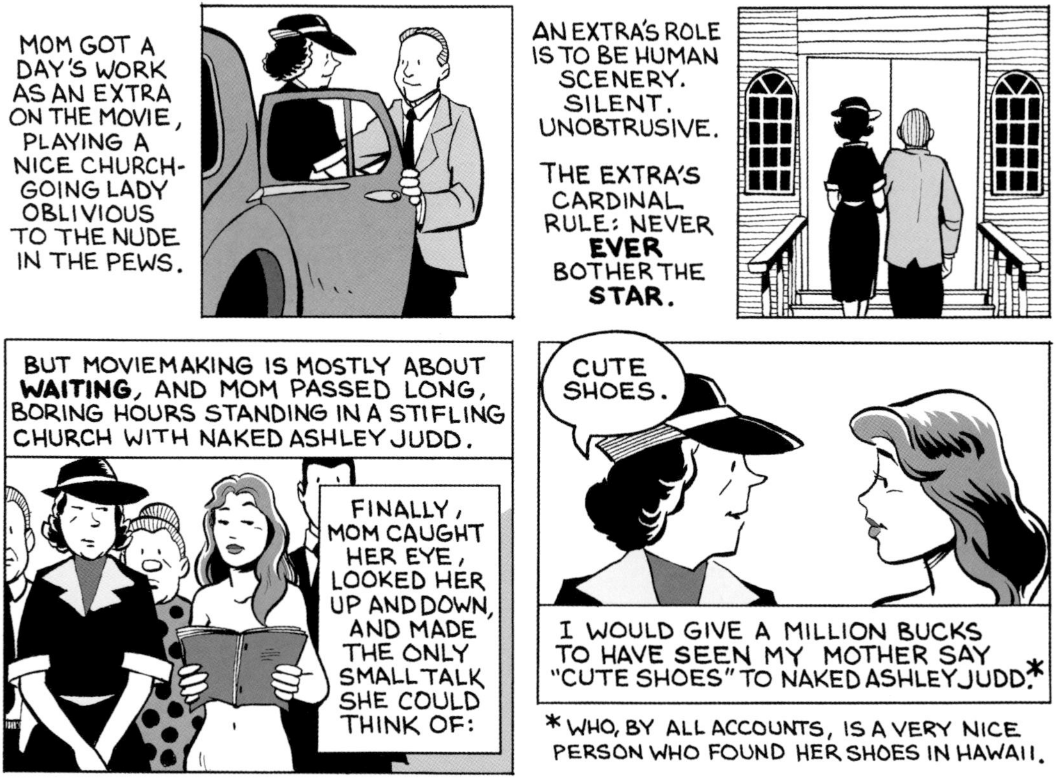
MOM GOT A DAY'S WORK AS AN EXTRA ON THE MOVIE, PLAYING A NICE CHURCH-GOING LADY OBLIVIOUS TO THE NUDE IN THE PEWS.
AN EXTRA'S ROLE IS TO BE HUMAN SCENERY. SILENT. UNOBTRUSIVE.
THE EXTRA'S CARDINAL RULE: NEVER **EVER** BOTHER THE **STAR**.
BUT MOVIEMAKING IS MOSTLY ABOUT **WAITING**, AND MOM PASSED LONG, BORING HOURS STANDING IN A STIFLING CHURCH WITH NAKED ASHLEY JUDD.
FINALLY, MOM CAUGHT HER EYE, LOOKED HER UP AND DOWN, AND MADE THE ONLY SMALL TALK SHE COULD THINK OF:
CUTE SHOES.
I WOULD GIVE A MILLION BUCKS TO HAVE SEEN MY MOTHER SAY "CUTE SHOES" TO NAKED ASHLEY JUDD.*
* WHO, BY ALL ACCOUNTS, IS A VERY NICE PERSON WHO FOUND HER SHOES IN HAWAII.

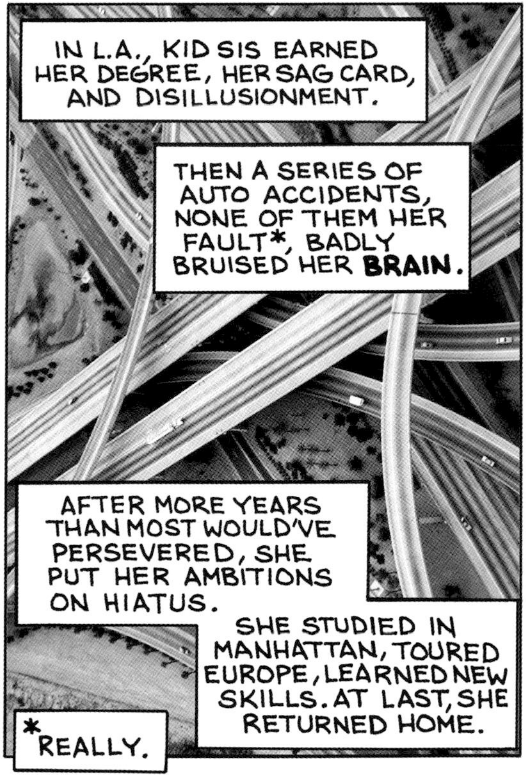
IN L.A., KID SIS EARNED HER DEGREE, HER SAG CARD, AND DISILLUSIONMENT.
THEN A SERIES OF AUTO ACCIDENTS, NONE OF THEM HER FAULT*, BADLY BRUISED HER **BRAIN**.
AFTER MORE YEARS THAN MOST WOULD'VE PERSEVERED, SHE PUT HER AMBITIONS ON HIATUS.
SHE STUDIED IN MANHATTAN, TOURED EUROPE, LEARNED NEW SKILLS. AT LAST, SHE RETURNED HOME.
*REALLY.

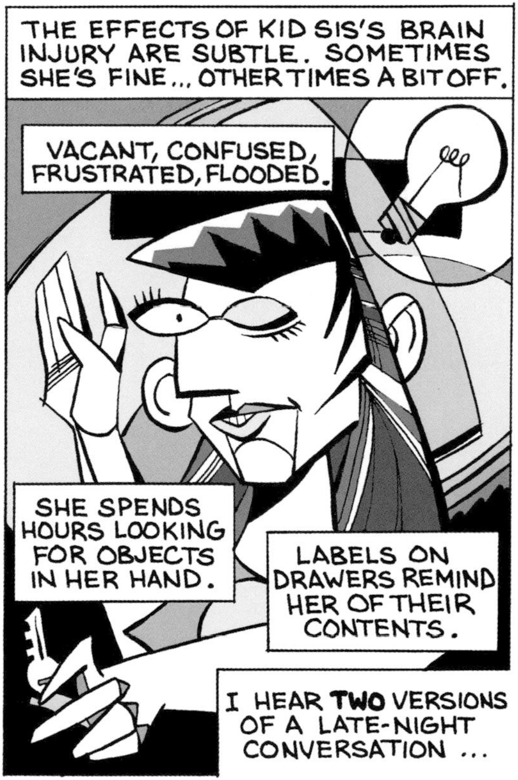
THE EFFECTS OF KID SIS'S BRAIN INJURY ARE SUBTLE. SOMETIMES SHE'S FINE... OTHER TIMES A BIT OFF.
VACANT, CONFUSED, FRUSTRATED, FLOODED.
SHE SPENDS HOURS LOOKING FOR OBJECTS IN HER HAND.
LABELS ON DRAWERS REMIND HER OF THEIR CONTENTS.
I HEAR **TWO** VERSIONS OF A LATE-NIGHT CONVERSATION ...

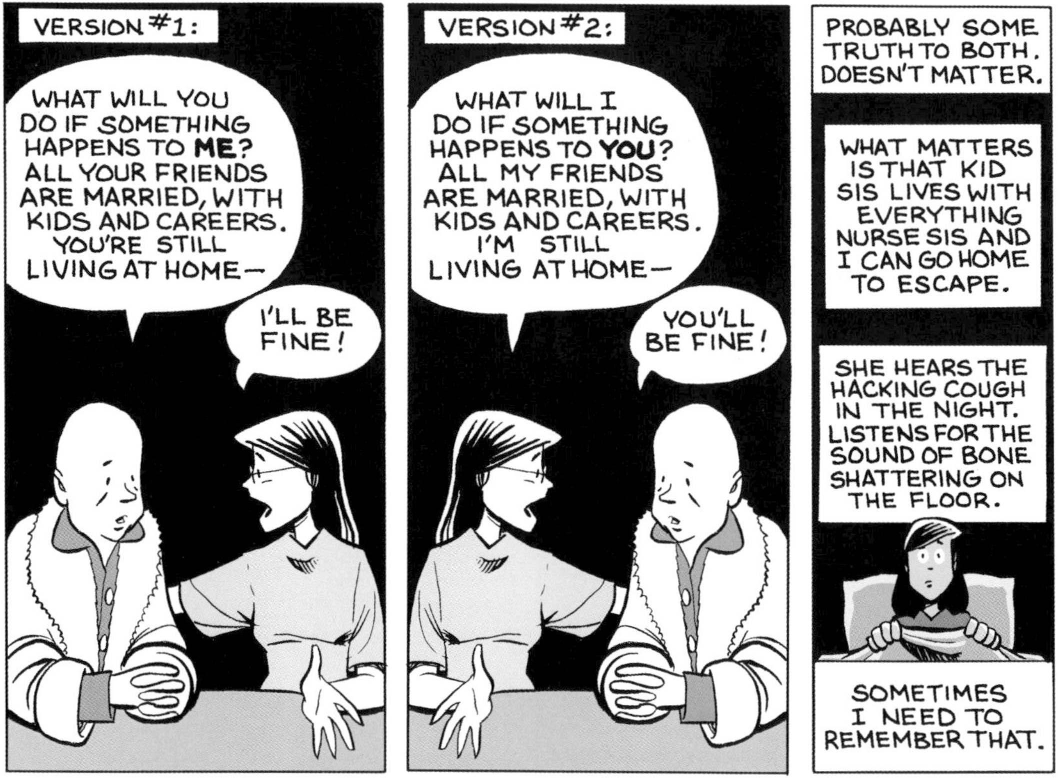
VERSION #1:
WHAT WILL YOU DO IF SOMETHING HAPPENS TO **ME**? ALL YOUR FRIENDS ARE MARRIED, WITH KIDS AND CAREERS. YOU'RE STILL LIVING AT HOME—
I'LL BE FINE!
VERSION #2:
WHAT WILL I DO IF SOMETHING HAPPENS TO **YOU**? ALL MY FRIENDS ARE MARRIED, WITH KIDS AND CAREERS. I'M STILL LIVING AT HOME—
YOU'LL BE FINE!
PROBABLY SOME TRUTH TO BOTH. DOESN'T MATTER.
WHAT MATTERS IS THAT KID SIS LIVES WITH EVERYTHING NURSE SIS AND I CAN GO HOME TO ESCAPE.
SHE HEARS THE HACKING COUGH IN THE NIGHT. LISTENS FOR THE SOUND OF BONE SHATTERING ON THE FLOOR.
SOMETIMES I NEED TO REMEMBER THAT.

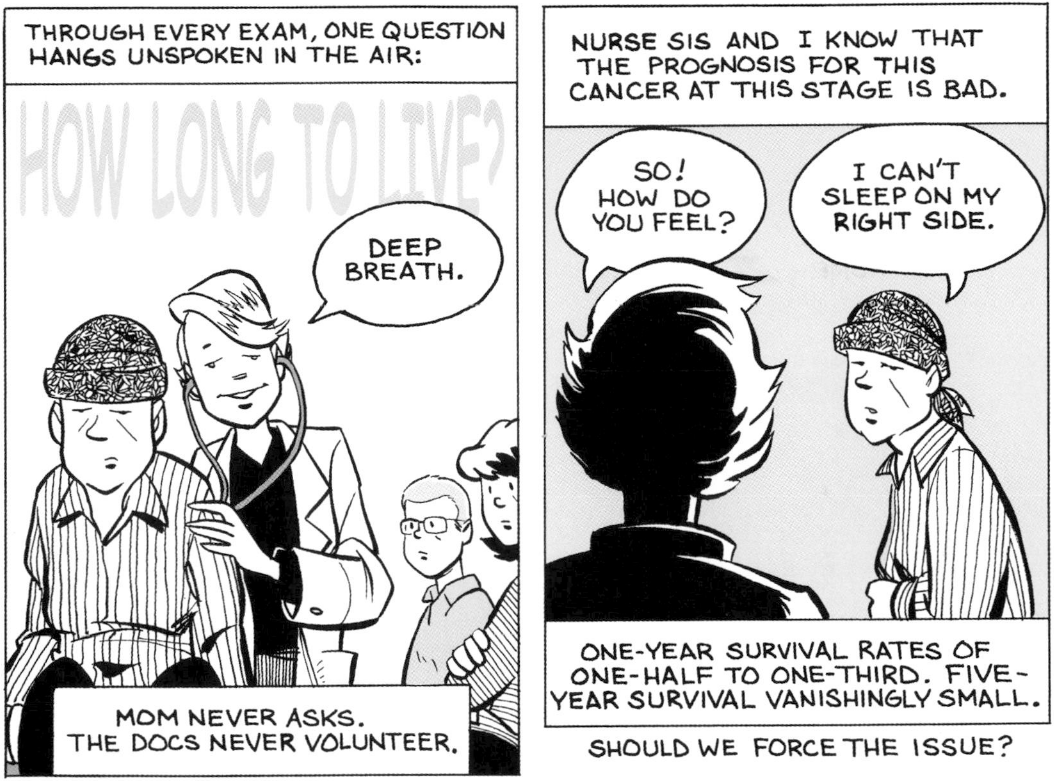
THROUGH EVERY EXAM, ONE QUESTION HANGS UNSPOKEN IN THE AIR:
HOW LONG TO LIVE?
DEEP BREATH.
MOM NEVER ASKS. THE DOCS NEVER VOLUNTEER.
NURSE SIS AND I KNOW THAT THE PROGNOSIS FOR THIS CANCER AT THIS STAGE IS BAD.
SO! HOW DO YOU FEEL?
I CAN'T SLEEP ON MY RIGHT SIDE.
ONE-YEAR SURVIVAL RATES OF ONE-HALF TO ONE-THIRD. FIVE-YEAR SURVIVAL VANISHINGLY SMALL.
SHOULD WE FORCE THE ISSUE?

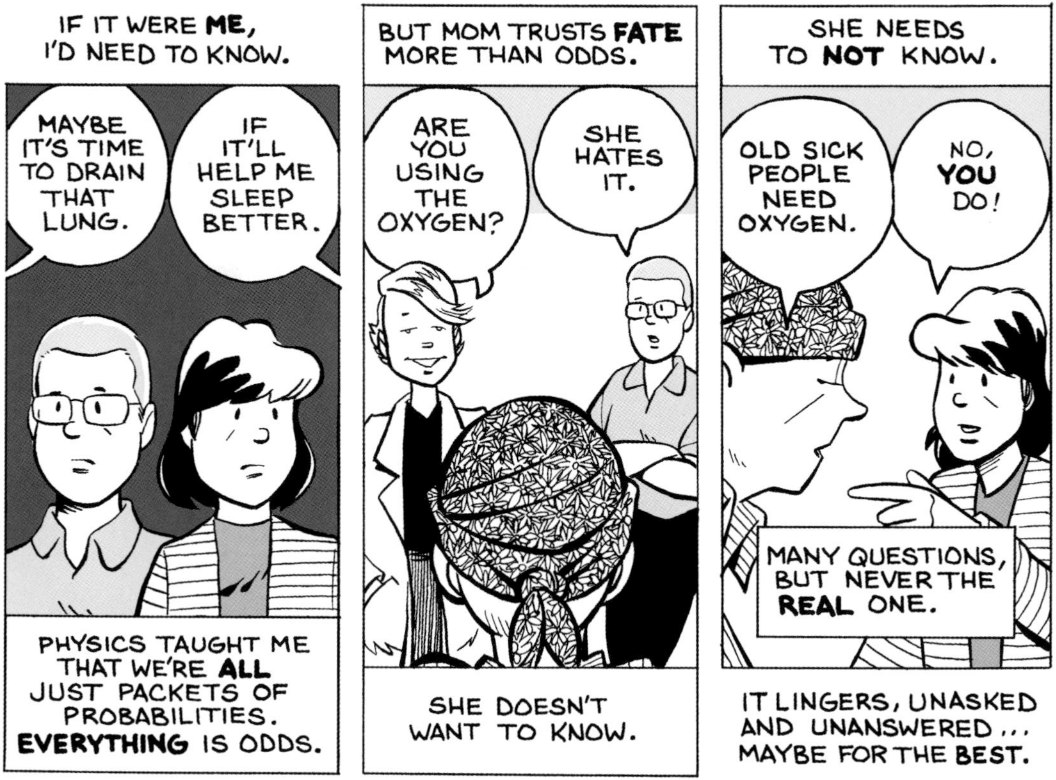
IF IT WERE **ME**, I'D NEED TO KNOW.
MAYBE IT'S TIME TO DRAIN THAT LUNG.
IF IT'LL HELP ME SLEEP BETTER.
PHYSICS TAUGHT ME THAT WE'RE **ALL** JUST PACKETS OF PROBABILITIES. **EVERYTHING** IS ODDS.
BUT MOM TRUSTS **FATE** MORE THAN ODDS.
ARE YOU USING THE OXYGEN?
SHE HATES IT.
SHE DOESN'T WANT TO KNOW.
SHE NEEDS TO **NOT** KNOW.
OLD SICK PEOPLE NEED OXYGEN.
NO, **YOU** DO!
MANY QUESTIONS, BUT NEVER THE **REAL** ONE.
IT LINGERS, UNASKED AND UNANSWERED... MAYBE FOR THE **BEST**.

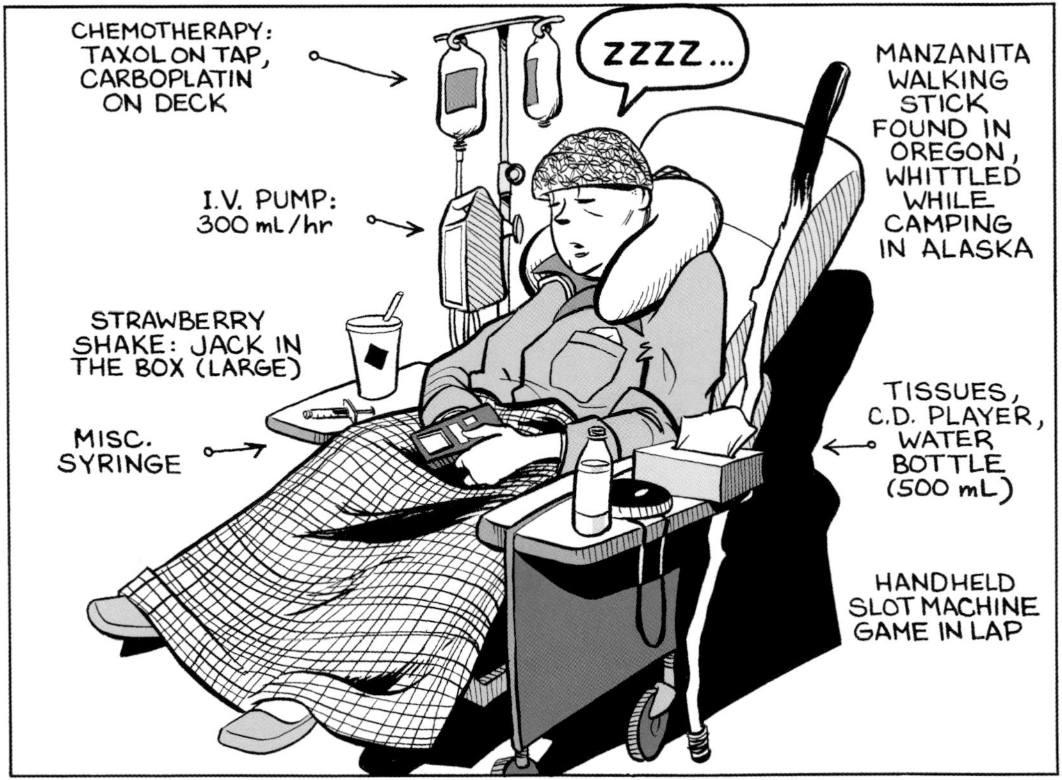
CHEMOTHERAPY: TAXOL ON TAP, CARBOPLATIN ON DECK
ZZZZ...
MANZANITA WALKING STICK FOUND IN OREGON, WHITTLED WHILE CAMPING IN ALASKA
I.V. PUMP: 300 mL/hr
STRAWBERRY SHAKE: JACK IN THE BOX (LARGE)
TISSUES, C.D. PLAYER, WATER BOTTLE (500 mL)
MISC. SYRINGE
HANDHELD SLOT MACHINE GAME IN LAP

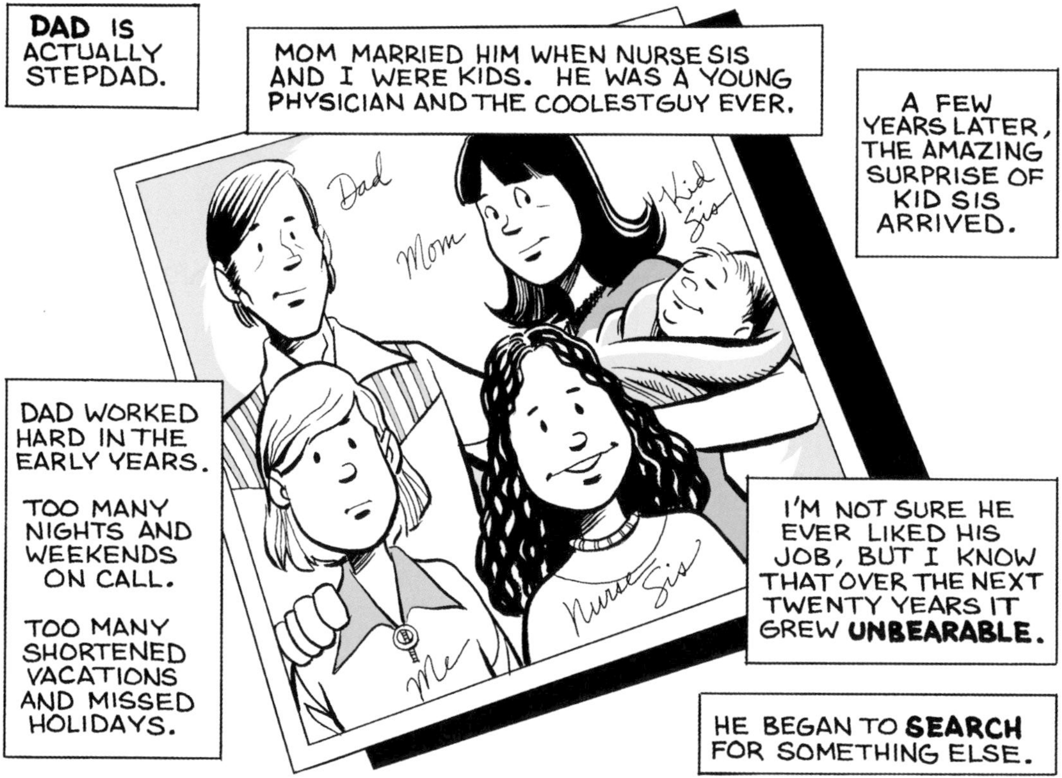
DAD IS ACTUALLY STEPDAD.
MOM MARRIED HIM WHEN NURSE SIS AND I WERE KIDS. HE WAS A YOUNG PHYSICIAN AND THE COOLEST GUY EVER.
A FEW YEARS LATER, THE AMAZING SURPRISE OF KID SIS ARRIVED.
Dad
Mom
Kid Sis
Me
Nurse Sis
DAD WORKED HARD IN THE EARLY YEARS.
TOO MANY NIGHTS AND WEEKENDS ON CALL.
TOO MANY SHORTENED VACATIONS AND MISSED HOLIDAYS.
I'M NOT SURE HE EVER LIKED HIS JOB, BUT I KNOW THAT OVER THE NEXT TWENTY YEARS IT GREW **UNBEARABLE**.
HE BEGAN TO **SEARCH** FOR SOMETHING ELSE.

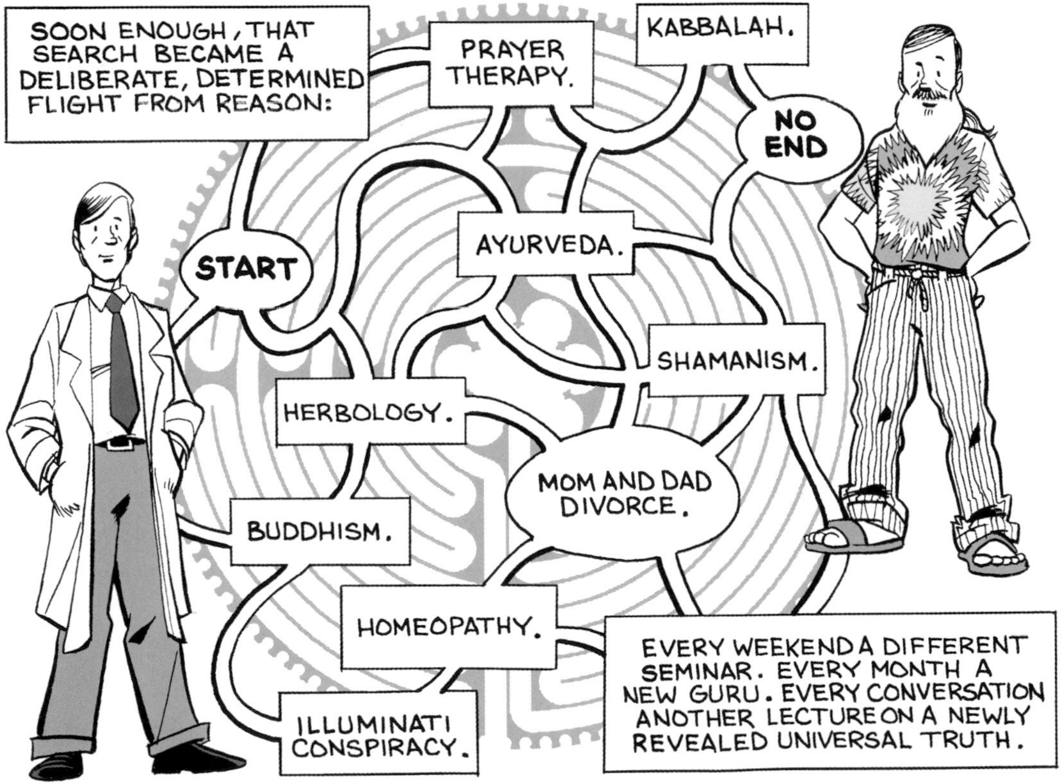
SOON ENOUGH, THAT SEARCH BECAME A DELIBERATE, DETERMINED FLIGHT FROM REASON:
START
PRAYER THERAPY.
KABBALAH.
NO END
AYURVEDA.
SHAMANISM.
HERBOLOGY.
MOM AND DAD DIVORCE.
BUDDHISM.
HOMEOPATHY.
ILLUMINATI CONSPIRACY.
EVERY WEEKEND A DIFFERENT SEMINAR. EVERY MONTH A NEW GURU. EVERY CONVERSATION ANOTHER LECTURE ON A NEWLY REVEALED UNIVERSAL TRUTH.

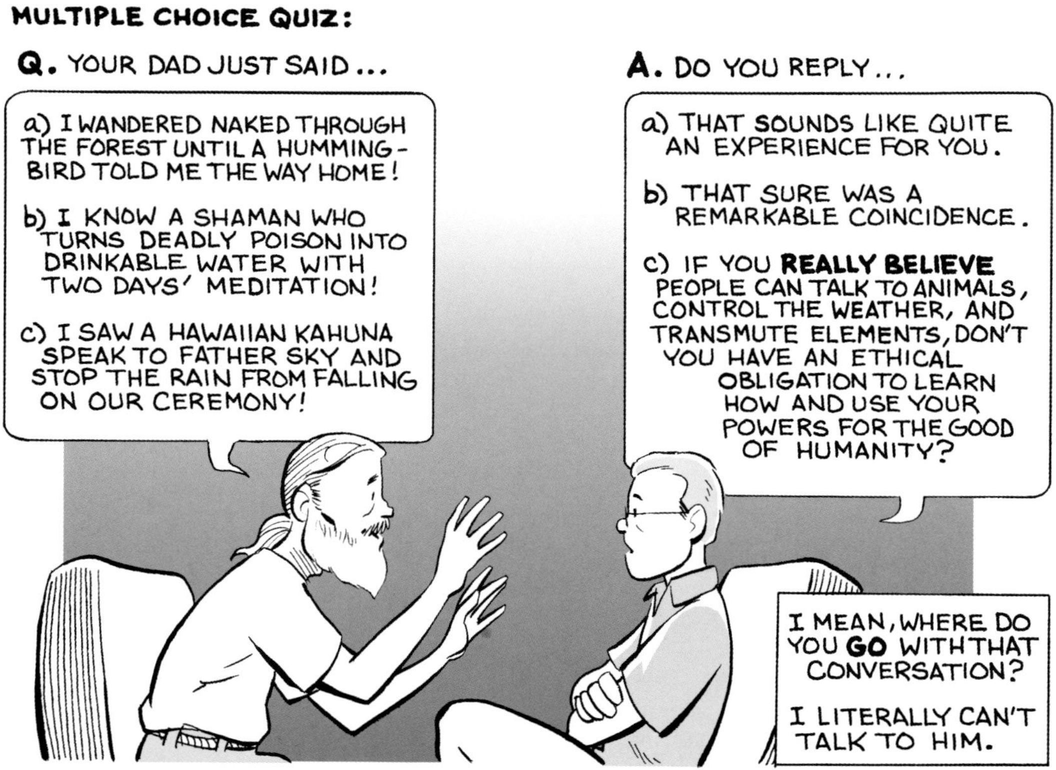
MULTIPLE CHOICE QUIZ:
Q. YOUR DAD JUST SAID...
a) I WANDERED NAKED THROUGH THE FOREST UNTIL A HUMMING-BIRD TOLD ME THE WAY HOME!
b) I KNOW A SHAMAN WHO TURNS DEADLY POISON INTO DRINKABLE WATER WITH TWO DAYS' MEDITATION!
c) I SAW A HAWAIIAN KAHUNA SPEAK TO FATHER SKY AND STOP THE RAIN FROM FALLING ON OUR CEREMONY!
A. DO YOU REPLY...
a) THAT SOUNDS LIKE QUITE AN EXPERIENCE FOR YOU.
b) THAT SURE WAS A REMARKABLE COINCIDENCE.
c) IF YOU **REALLY BELIEVE** PEOPLE CAN TALK TO ANIMALS, CONTROL THE WEATHER, AND TRANSMUTE ELEMENTS, DON'T YOU HAVE AN ETHICAL OBLIGATION TO LEARN HOW AND USE YOUR POWERS FOR THE GOOD OF HUMANITY?
I MEAN, WHERE DO YOU **GO** WITH THAT CONVERSATION?
I LITERALLY CAN'T TALK TO HIM.

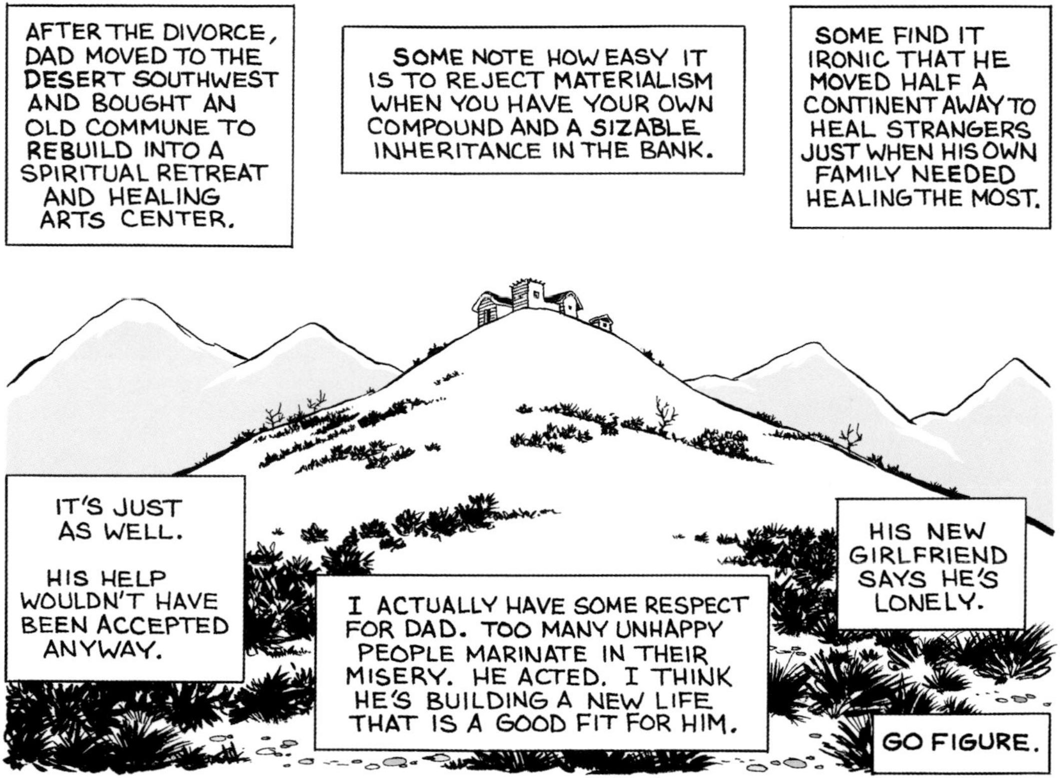
AFTER THE DIVORCE, DAD MOVED TO THE DESERT SOUTHWEST AND BOUGHT AN OLD COMMUNE TO REBUILD INTO A SPIRITUAL RETREAT AND HEALING ARTS CENTER.
SOME NOTE HOW EASY IT IS TO REJECT MATERIALISM WHEN YOU HAVE YOUR OWN COMPOUND AND A SIZABLE INHERITANCE IN THE BANK.
SOME FIND IT IRONIC THAT HE MOVED HALF A CONTINENT AWAY TO HEAL STRANGERS JUST WHEN HIS OWN FAMILY NEEDED HEALING THE MOST.
IT'S JUST AS WELL.
HIS HELP WOULDN'T HAVE BEEN ACCEPTED ANYWAY.
I ACTUALLY HAVE SOME RESPECT FOR DAD. TOO MANY UNHAPPY PEOPLE MARINATE IN THEIR MISERY. HE ACTED. I THINK HE'S BUILDING A NEW LIFE THAT IS A GOOD FIT FOR HIM.
HIS NEW GIRLFRIEND SAYS HE'S LONELY.
GO FIGURE.

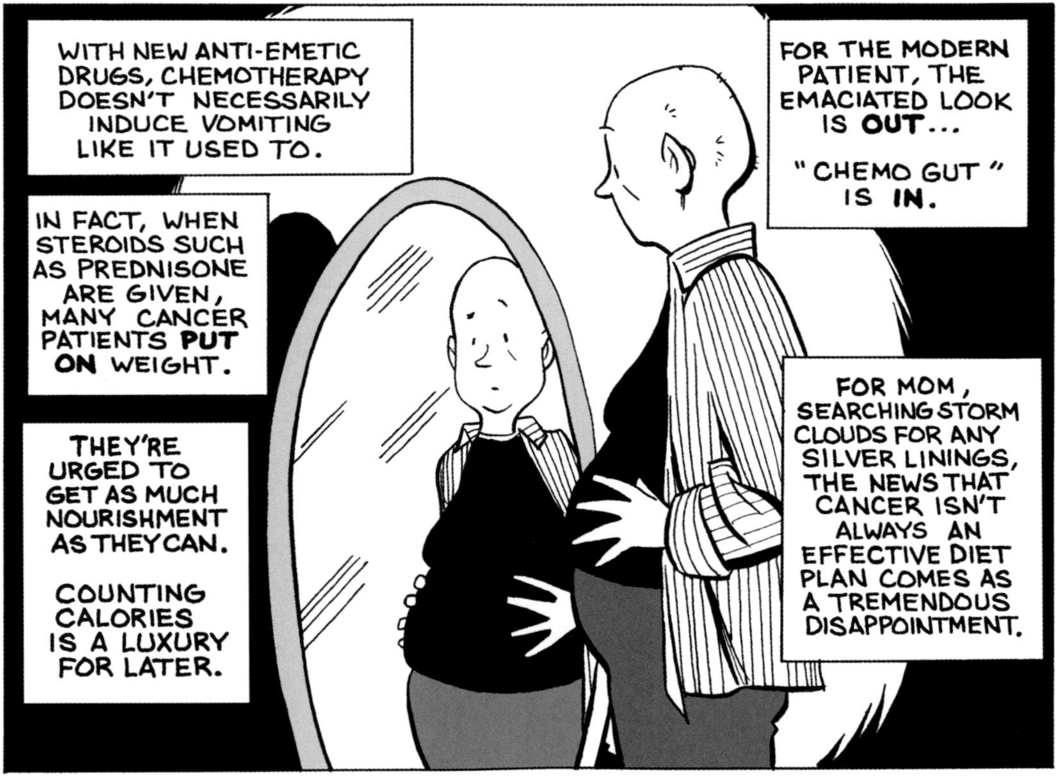
WITH NEW ANTI-EMETIC DRUGS, CHEMOTHERAPY DOESN'T NECESSARILY INDUCE VOMITING LIKE IT USED TO.
IN FACT, WHEN STEROIDS SUCH AS PREDNISONE ARE GIVEN, MANY CANCER PATIENTS **PUT ON** WEIGHT.
THEY'RE URGED TO GET AS MUCH NOURISHMENT AS THEY CAN.
COUNTING CALORIES IS A LUXURY FOR LATER.
FOR THE MODERN PATIENT, THE EMACIATED LOOK IS **OUT**...
"CHEMO GUT" IS **IN**.
FOR MOM, SEARCHING STORM CLOUDS FOR ANY SILVER LININGS, THE NEWS THAT CANCER ISN'T ALWAYS AN EFFECTIVE DIET PLAN COMES AS A TREMENDOUS DISAPPOINTMENT.

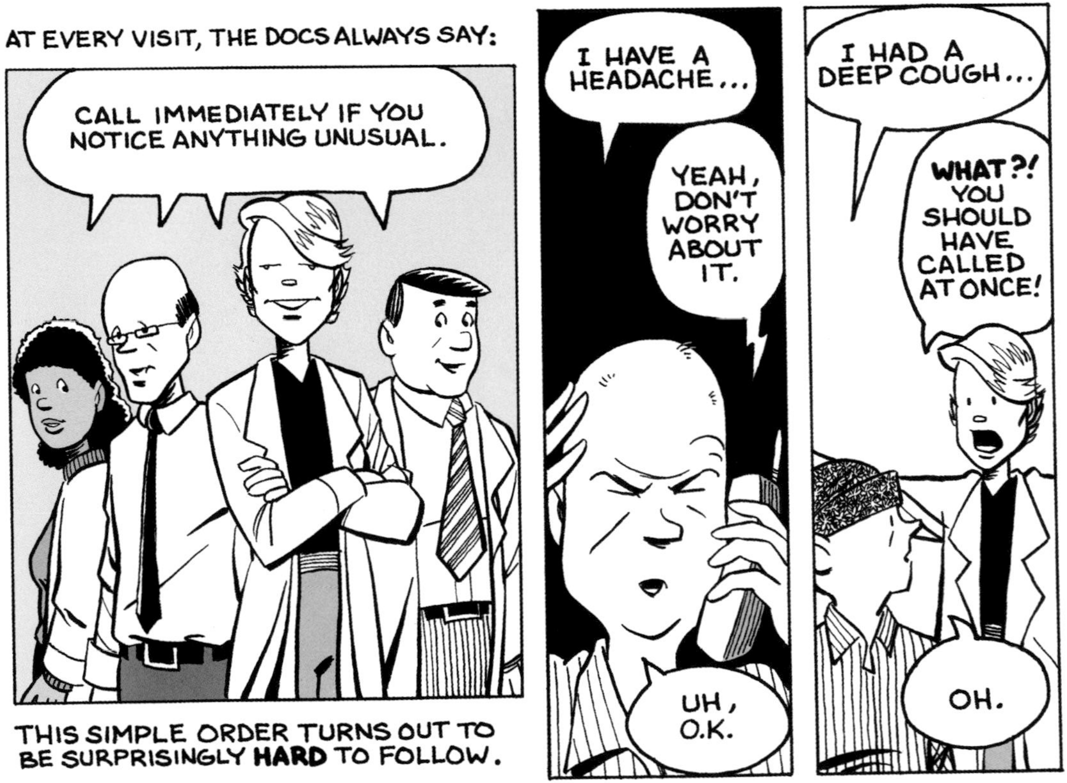
AT EVERY VISIT, THE DOCS ALWAYS SAY:
CALL IMMEDIATELY IF YOU NOTICE ANYTHING UNUSUAL.
THIS SIMPLE ORDER TURNS OUT TO BE SURPRISINGLY **HARD** TO FOLLOW.
I HAVE A HEADACHE...
YEAH, DON'T WORRY ABOUT IT.
UH, O.K.
I HAD A DEEP COUGH...
WHAT?! YOU SHOULD HAVE CALLED AT ONCE!
OH.

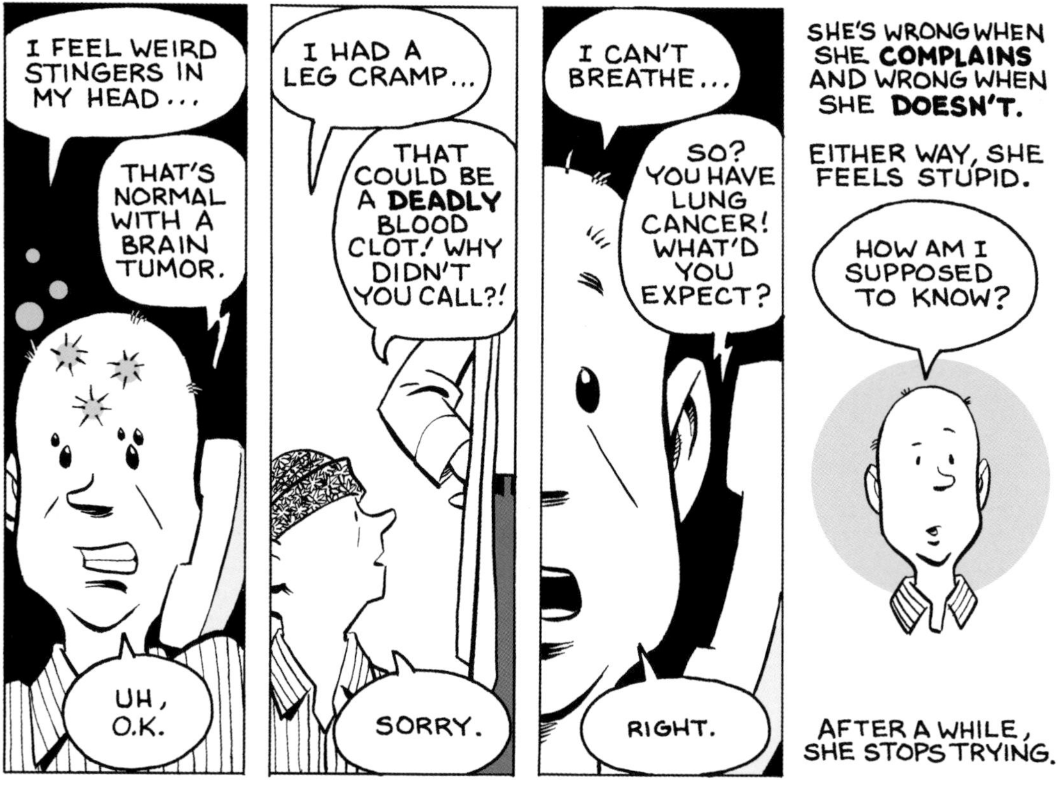
I FEEL WEIRD STINGERS IN MY HEAD...
THAT'S NORMAL WITH A BRAIN TUMOR.
UH, O.K.
I HAD A LEG CRAMP...
THAT COULD BE A **DEADLY** BLOOD CLOT! WHY DIDN'T YOU CALL?!
SORRY.
I CAN'T BREATHE...
SO? YOU HAVE LUNG CANCER! WHAT'D YOU EXPECT?
RIGHT.
SHE'S WRONG WHEN SHE **COMPLAINS** AND WRONG WHEN SHE **DOESN'T.**
EITHER WAY, SHE FEELS STUPID.
HOW AM I SUPPOSED TO KNOW?
AFTER A WHILE, SHE STOPS TRYING.

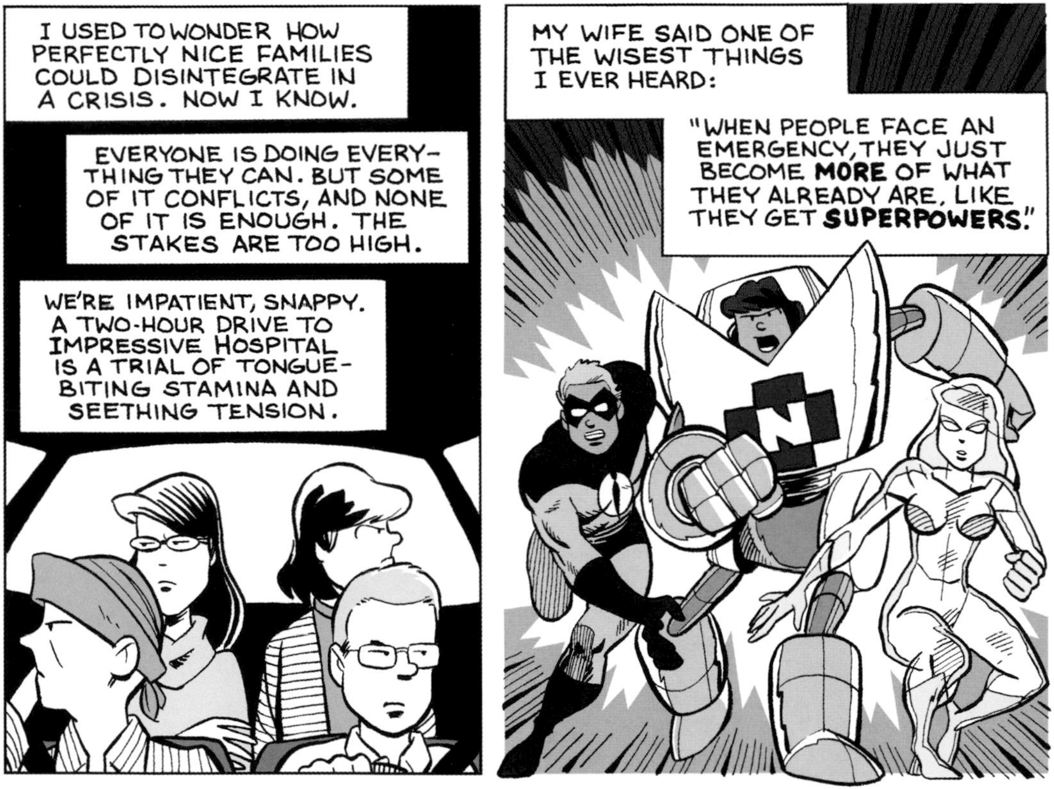
I USED TO WONDER HOW PERFECTLY NICE FAMILIES COULD DISINTEGRATE IN A CRISIS. NOW I KNOW.
EVERYONE IS DOING EVERYTHING THEY CAN. BUT SOME OF IT CONFLICTS, AND NONE OF IT IS ENOUGH. THE STAKES ARE TOO HIGH.
WE'RE IMPATIENT, SNAPPY. A TWO-HOUR DRIVE TO IMPRESSIVE HOSPITAL IS A TRIAL OF TONGUE-BITING STAMINA AND SEETHING TENSION.
MY WIFE SAID ONE OF THE WISEST THINGS I EVER HEARD:
"WHEN PEOPLE FACE AN EMERGENCY, THEY JUST BECOME **MORE** OF WHAT THEY ALREADY ARE, LIKE THEY GET **SUPERPOWERS**."
N

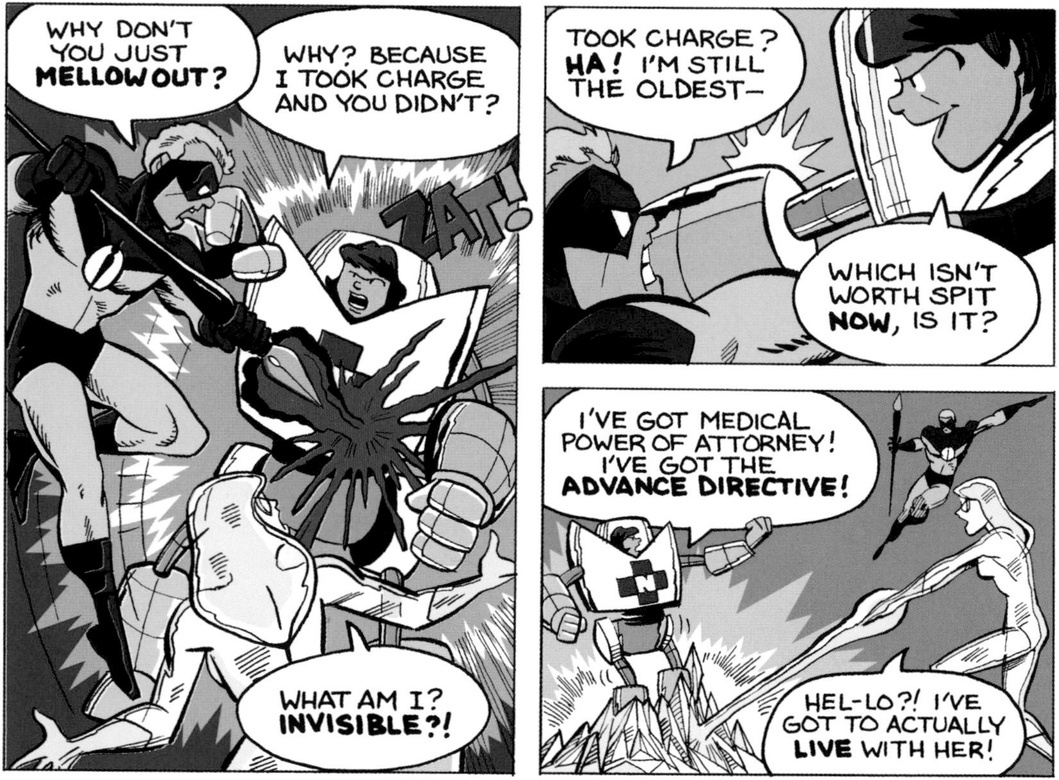
WHY DON'T YOU JUST MELLOW OUT?
WHY? BECAUSE I TOOK CHARGE AND YOU DIDN'T?
ZAT!
WHAT AM I? INVISIBLE?!
TOOK CHARGE? HA! I'M STILL THE OLDEST—
WHICH ISN'T WORTH SPIT NOW, IS IT?
I'VE GOT MEDICAL POWER OF ATTORNEY! I'VE GOT THE ADVANCE DIRECTIVE!
HEL-LO?! I'VE GOT TO ACTUALLY LIVE WITH HER!

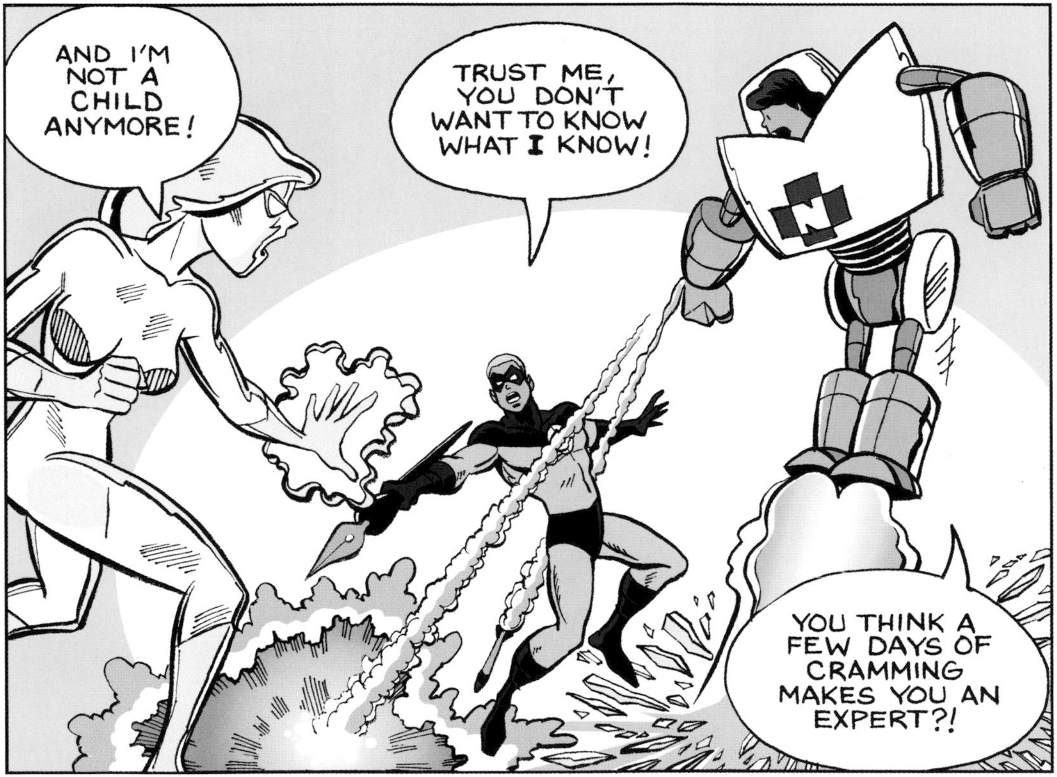
AND I'M NOT A CHILD ANYMORE!
TRUST ME, YOU DON'T WANT TO KNOW WHAT I KNOW!
YOU THINK A FEW DAYS OF CRAMMING MAKES YOU AN EXPERT?!

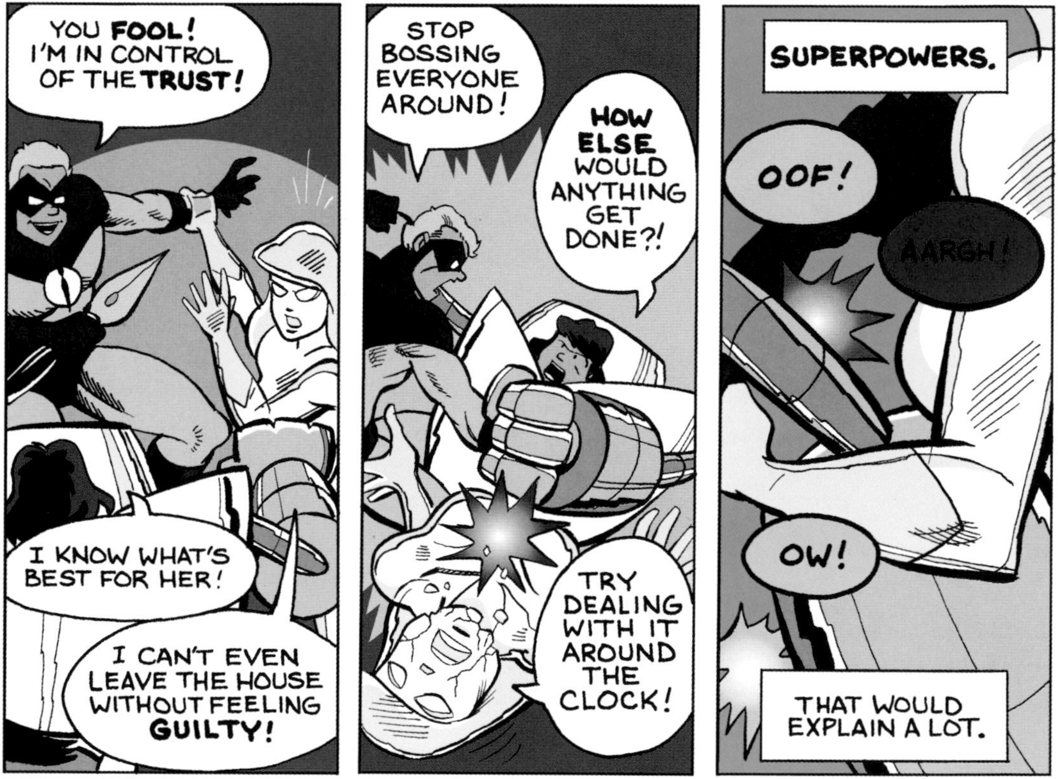
YOU **FOOL**! I'M IN CONTROL OF THE **TRUST**!
I KNOW WHAT'S BEST FOR HER!
I CAN'T EVEN LEAVE THE HOUSE WITHOUT FEELING **GUILTY**!
STOP BOSSING EVERYONE AROUND!
HOW ELSE WOULD ANYTHING GET DONE?!
TRY DEALING WITH IT AROUND THE CLOCK!
SUPERPOWERS.
OOF!
AARGH!
OW!
THAT WOULD EXPLAIN A LOT.

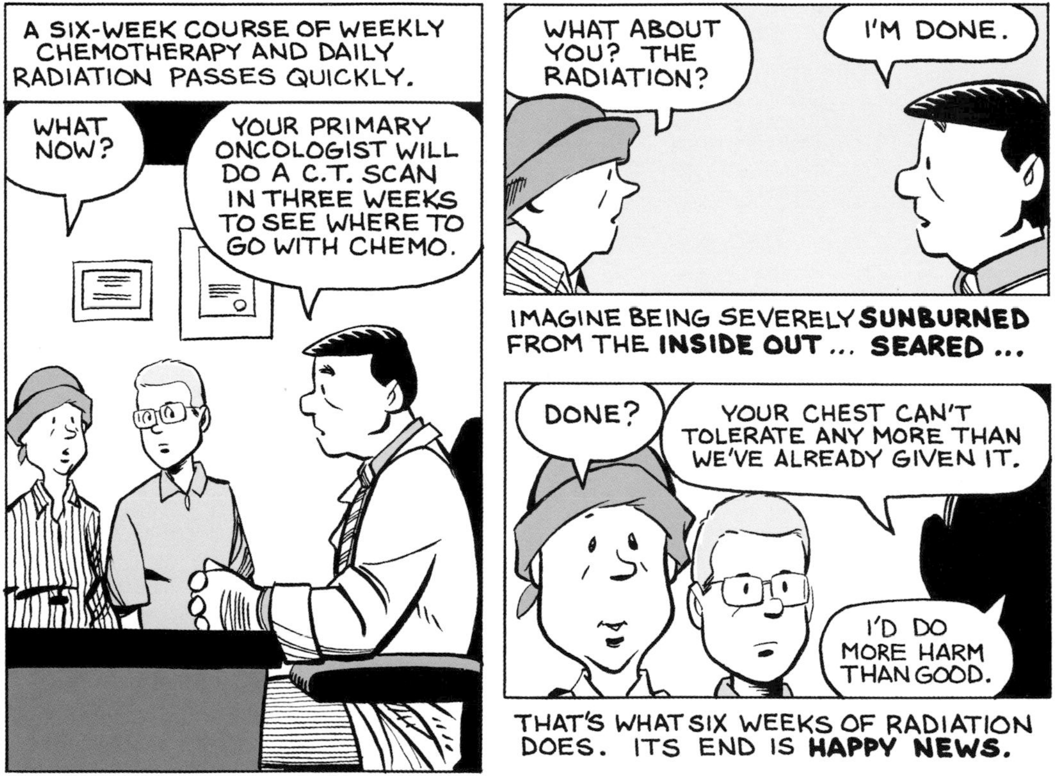
A SIX-WEEK COURSE OF WEEKLY CHEMOTHERAPY AND DAILY RADIATION PASSES QUICKLY.
WHAT NOW?
YOUR PRIMARY ONCOLOGIST WILL DO A C.T. SCAN IN THREE WEEKS TO SEE WHERE TO GO WITH CHEMO.
WHAT ABOUT YOU? THE RADIATION?
I'M DONE.
IMAGINE BEING SEVERELY **SUNBURNED** FROM THE **INSIDE OUT** ... **SEARED** ...
DONE?
YOUR CHEST CAN'T TOLERATE ANY MORE THAN WE'VE ALREADY GIVEN IT.
I'D DO MORE HARM THAN GOOD.
THAT'S WHAT SIX WEEKS OF RADIATION DOES. ITS END IS **HAPPY NEWS.**

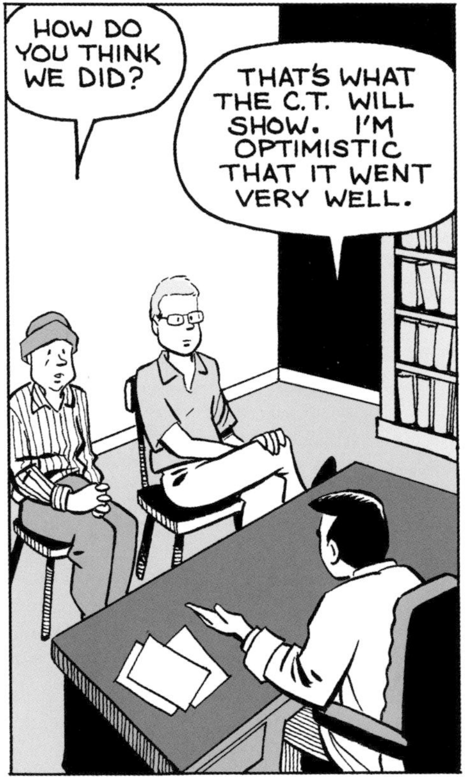
HOW DO YOU THINK WE DID?
THAT'S WHAT THE C.T. WILL SHOW. I'M OPTIMISTIC THAT IT WENT VERY WELL.

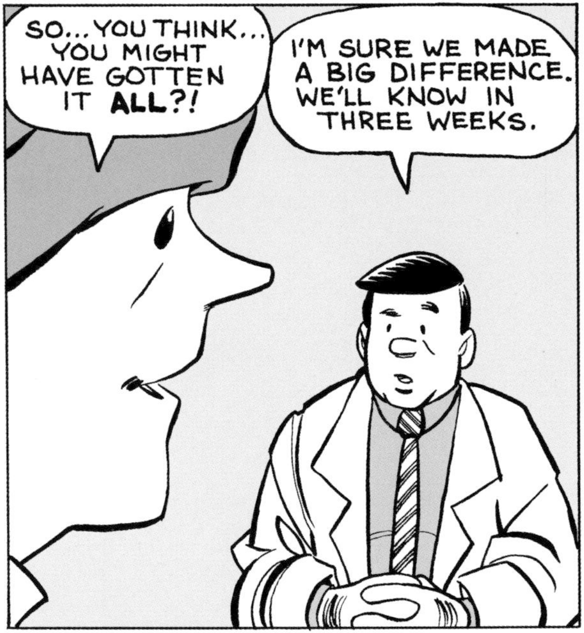
SO... YOU THINK... YOU MIGHT HAVE GOTTEN IT **ALL**?!
I'M SURE WE MADE A BIG DIFFERENCE. WE'LL KNOW IN THREE WEEKS.

MOM HEARS ONLY WHAT SHE WANTS TO— **NEEDS TO**—HEAR. SHE DOESN'T CATCH THE REST: EITHER WAY, THERE'S NOTHING MORE HE CAN DO.

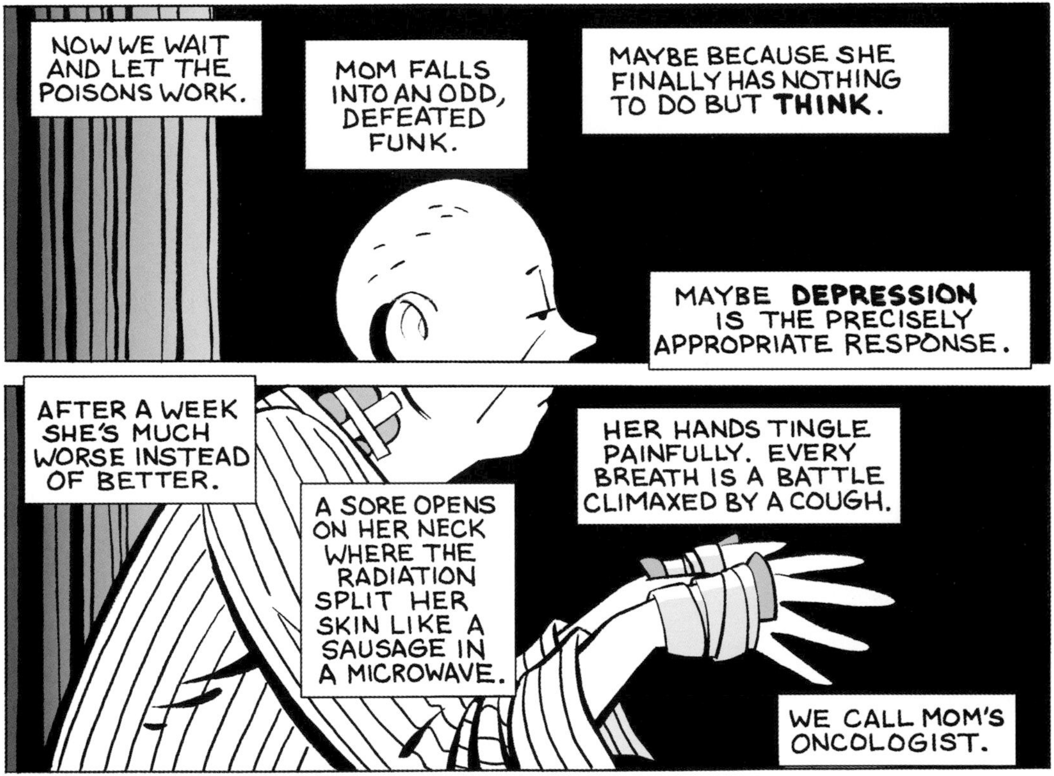
NOW WE WAIT AND LET THE POISONS WORK.
MOM FALLS INTO AN ODD, DEFEATED FUNK.
MAYBE BECAUSE SHE FINALLY HAS NOTHING TO DO BUT **THINK**.
MAYBE **DEPRESSION** IS THE PRECISELY APPROPRIATE RESPONSE.
AFTER A WEEK SHE'S MUCH WORSE INSTEAD OF BETTER.
A SORE OPENS ON HER NECK WHERE THE RADIATION SPLIT HER SKIN LIKE A SAUSAGE IN A MICROWAVE.
HER HANDS TINGLE PAINFULLY. EVERY BREATH IS A BATTLE CLIMAXED BY A COUGH.
WE CALL MOM'S ONCOLOGIST.

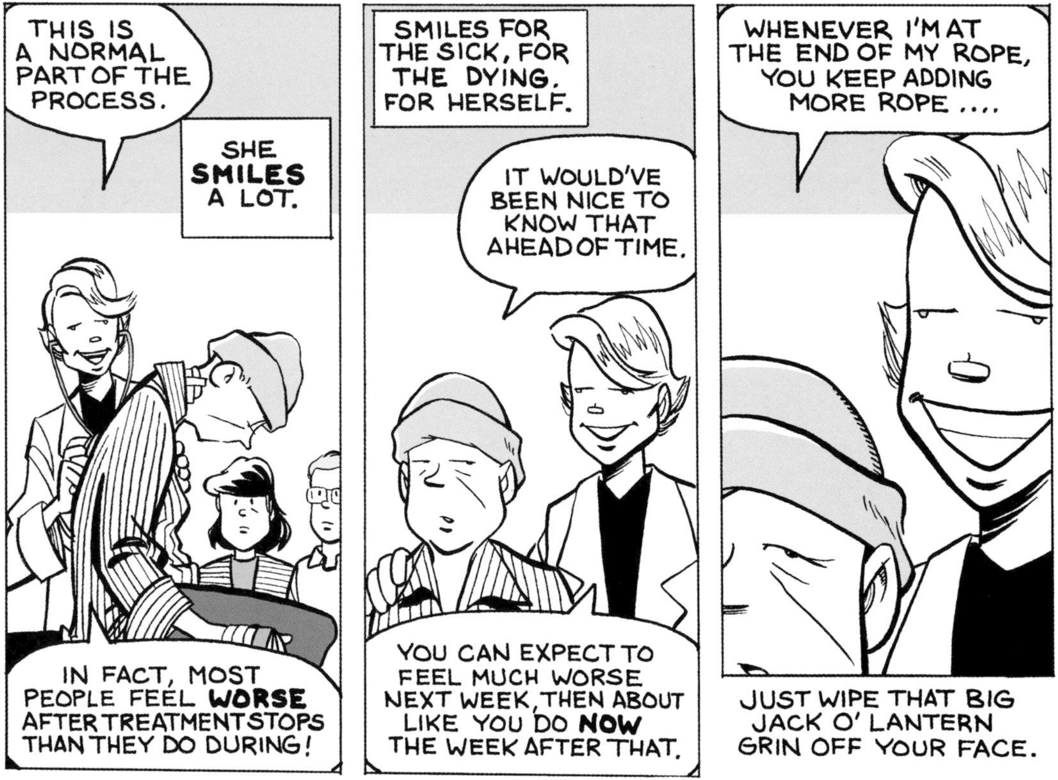
THIS IS A NORMAL PART OF THE PROCESS.
SHE **SMILES** A LOT.
IN FACT, MOST PEOPLE FEEL **WORSE** AFTER TREATMENT STOPS THAN THEY DO DURING!
SMILES FOR THE SICK, FOR THE DYING, FOR HERSELF.
IT WOULD'VE BEEN NICE TO KNOW THAT AHEAD OF TIME.
YOU CAN EXPECT TO FEEL MUCH WORSE NEXT WEEK, THEN ABOUT LIKE YOU DO **NOW** THE WEEK AFTER THAT.
WHENEVER I'M AT THE END OF MY ROPE, YOU KEEP ADDING MORE ROPE ....
JUST WIPE THAT BIG JACK O' LANTERN GRIN OFF YOUR FACE.

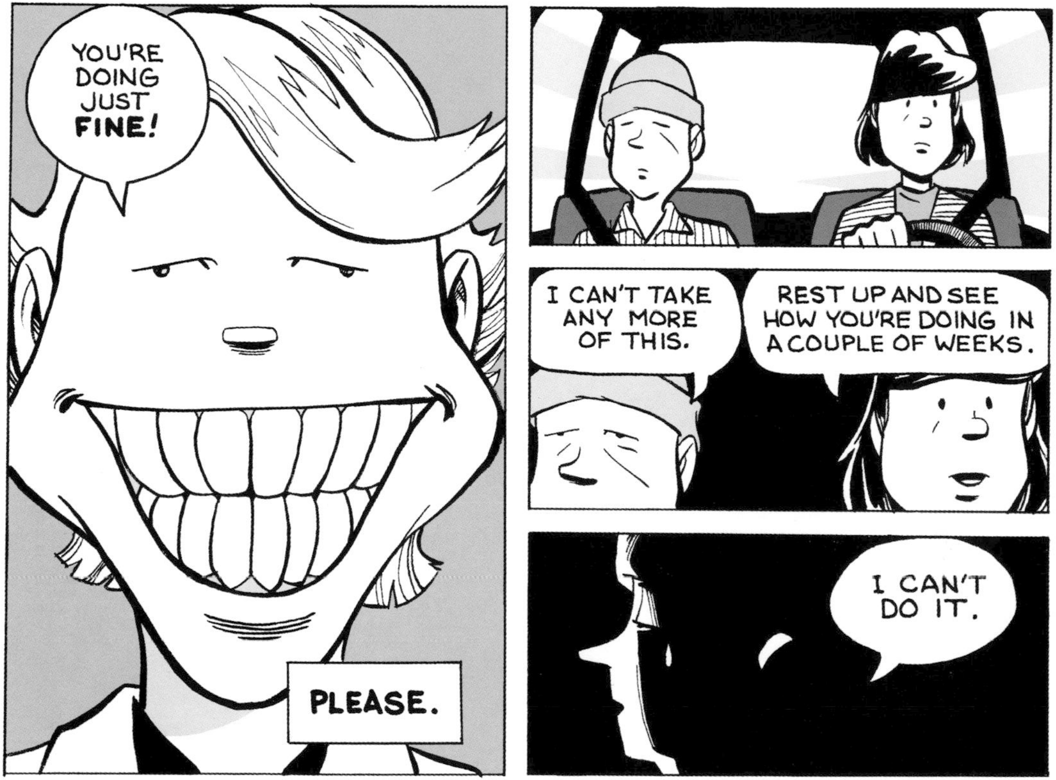
YOU'RE DOING JUST FINE!
PLEASE.
I CAN'T TAKE ANY MORE OF THIS.
REST UP AND SEE HOW YOU'RE DOING IN A COUPLE OF WEEKS.
I CAN'T DO IT.

AFTER THE WAR, PART ONE

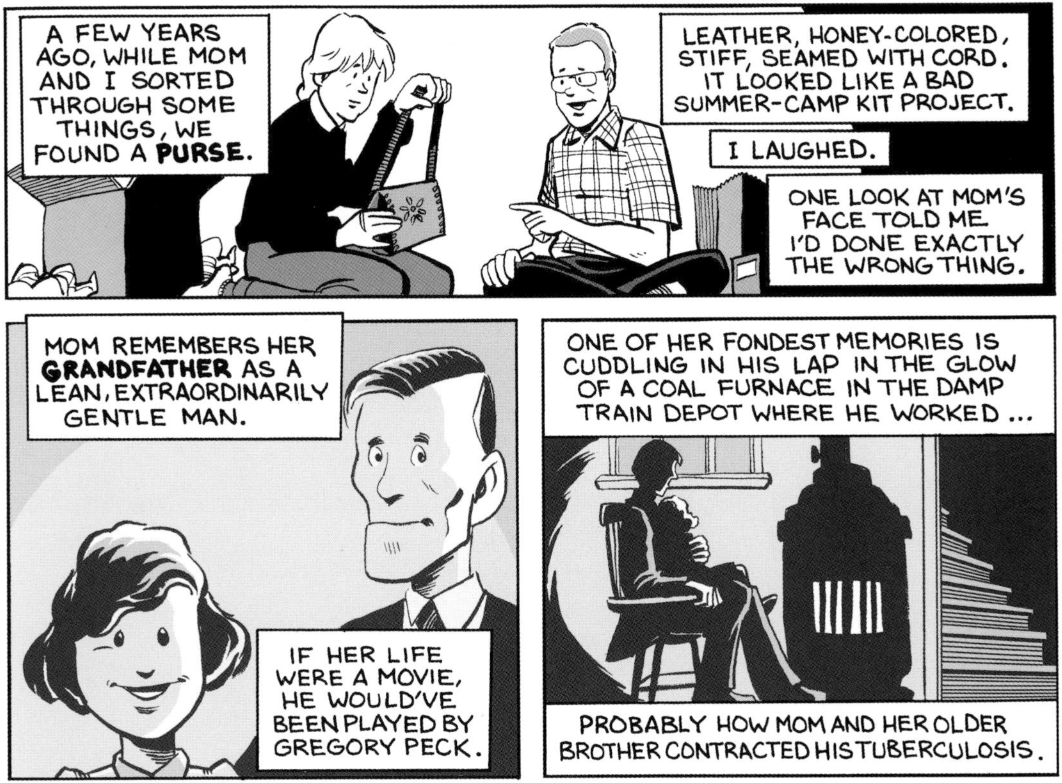
A FEW YEARS AGO, WHILE MOM AND I SORTED THROUGH SOME THINGS, WE FOUND A **PURSE**.
LEATHER, HONEY-COLORED, STIFF, SEAMED WITH CORD. IT LOOKED LIKE A BAD SUMMER-CAMP KIT PROJECT.
I LAUGHED.
ONE LOOK AT MOM'S FACE TOLD ME I'D DONE EXACTLY THE WRONG THING.
MOM REMEMBERS HER **GRANDFATHER** AS A LEAN, EXTRAORDINARILY GENTLE MAN.
IF HER LIFE WERE A MOVIE, HE WOULD'VE BEEN PLAYED BY GREGORY PECK.
ONE OF HER FONDEST MEMORIES IS CUDDLING IN HIS LAP IN THE GLOW OF A COAL FURNACE IN THE DAMP TRAIN DEPOT WHERE HE WORKED ...
PROBABLY HOW MOM AND HER OLDER BROTHER CONTRACTED HIS TUBERCULOSIS.

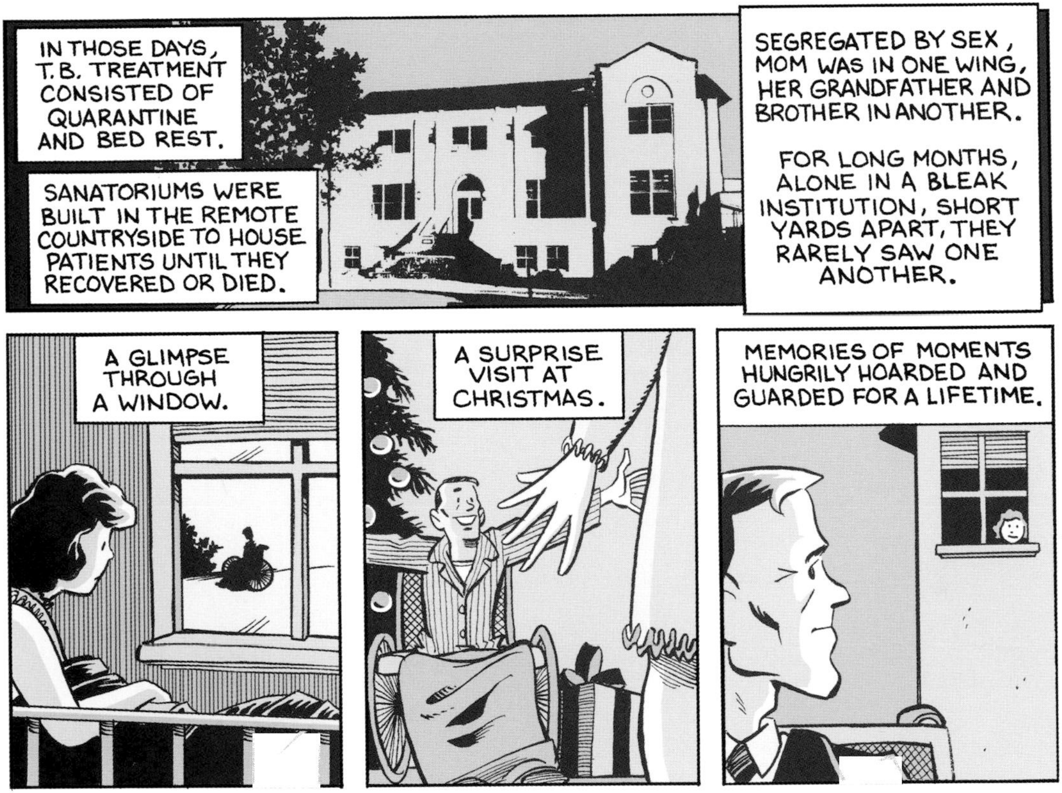
IN THOSE DAYS, T.B. TREATMENT CONSISTED OF QUARANTINE AND BED REST.
SANATORIUMS WERE BUILT IN THE REMOTE COUNTRYSIDE TO HOUSE PATIENTS UNTIL THEY RECOVERED OR DIED.
SEGREGATED BY SEX, MOM WAS IN ONE WING, HER GRANDFATHER AND BROTHER IN ANOTHER.
FOR LONG MONTHS, ALONE IN A BLEAK INSTITUTION, SHORT YARDS APART, THEY RARELY SAW ONE ANOTHER.
A GLIMPSE THROUGH A WINDOW.
A SURPRISE VISIT AT CHRISTMAS.
MEMORIES OF MOMENTS HUNGRILY HOARDED AND GUARDED FOR A LIFETIME.

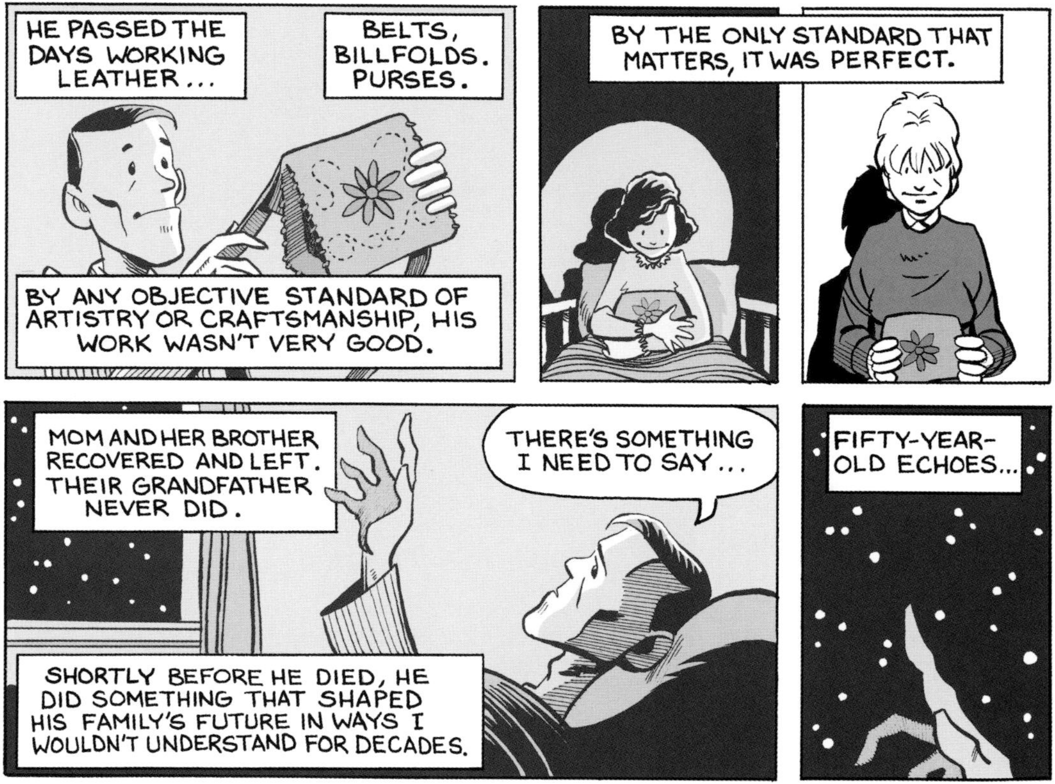
HE PASSED THE DAYS WORKING LEATHER...
BELTS, BILLFOLDS. PURSES.
BY ANY OBJECTIVE STANDARD OF ARTISTRY OR CRAFTSMANSHIP, HIS WORK WASN'T VERY GOOD.
BY THE ONLY STANDARD THAT MATTERS, IT WAS PERFECT.
MOM AND HER BROTHER RECOVERED AND LEFT. THEIR GRANDFATHER NEVER DID.
THERE'S SOMETHING I NEED TO SAY...
SHORTLY BEFORE HE DIED, HE DID SOMETHING THAT SHAPED HIS FAMILY'S FUTURE IN WAYS I WOULDN'T UNDERSTAND FOR DECADES.
FIFTY-YEAR-OLD ECHOES...

ONE DIMENSION:
LINE A IS **2 TIMES** AS LONG AS LINE B.

A
B

TWO DIMENSIONS:
AREA VARIES WITH THE SQUARE OF LENGTH. THE AREA OF SQUARE A IS 2^2 = **4 TIMES** THAT OF SQUARE B.

A
B

THREE DIMENSIONS:
VOLUME VARIES WITH THE CUBE OF LENGTH. THE VOLUME OF CUBE A IS 2^3 = **8 TIMES** THAT OF CUBE B.

A
B

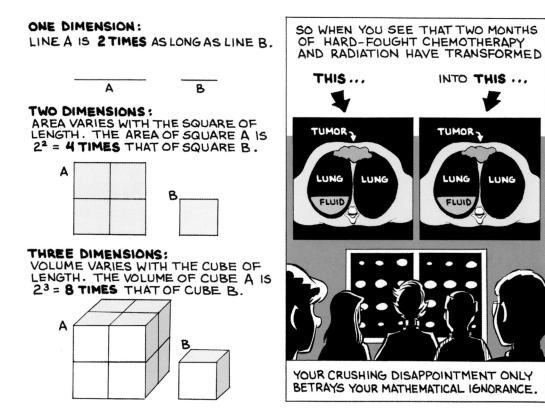

SO WHEN YOU SEE THAT TWO MONTHS OF HARD-FOUGHT CHEMOTHERAPY AND RADIATION HAVE TRANSFORMED
THIS...
INTO THIS...
TUMOR
LUNG
LUNG
FLUID
TUMOR
LUNG
LUNG
FLUID
YOUR CRUSHING DISAPPOINTMENT ONLY BETRAYS YOUR MATHEMATICAL IGNORANCE.

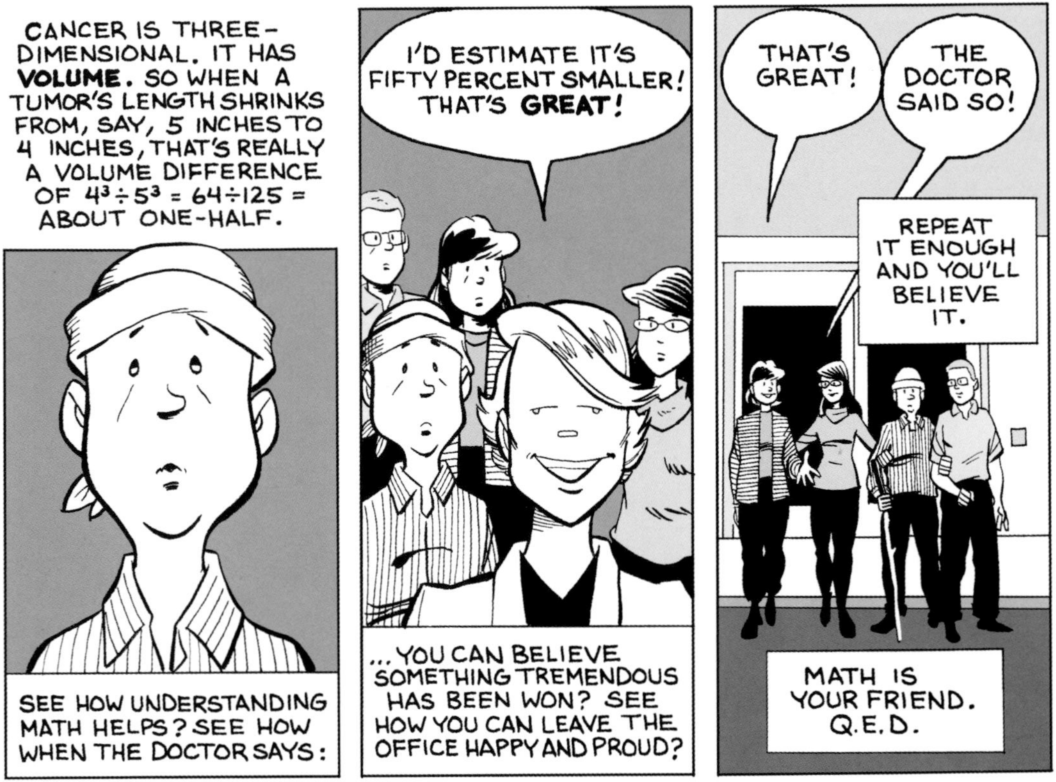
CANCER IS THREE-DIMENSIONAL. IT HAS **VOLUME.** SO WHEN A TUMOR'S LENGTH SHRINKS FROM, SAY, 5 INCHES TO 4 INCHES, THAT'S REALLY A VOLUME DIFFERENCE OF $4^3 \div 5^3 = 64 \div 125 =$ ABOUT ONE-HALF.
SEE HOW UNDERSTANDING MATH HELPS? SEE HOW WHEN THE DOCTOR SAYS:
I'D ESTIMATE IT'S FIFTY PERCENT SMALLER! THAT'S **GREAT!**
...YOU CAN BELIEVE SOMETHING TREMENDOUS HAS BEEN WON? SEE HOW YOU CAN LEAVE THE OFFICE HAPPY AND PROUD?
THAT'S GREAT!
THE DOCTOR SAID SO!
REPEAT IT ENOUGH AND YOU'LL BELIEVE IT.
MATH IS YOUR FRIEND. Q.E.D.

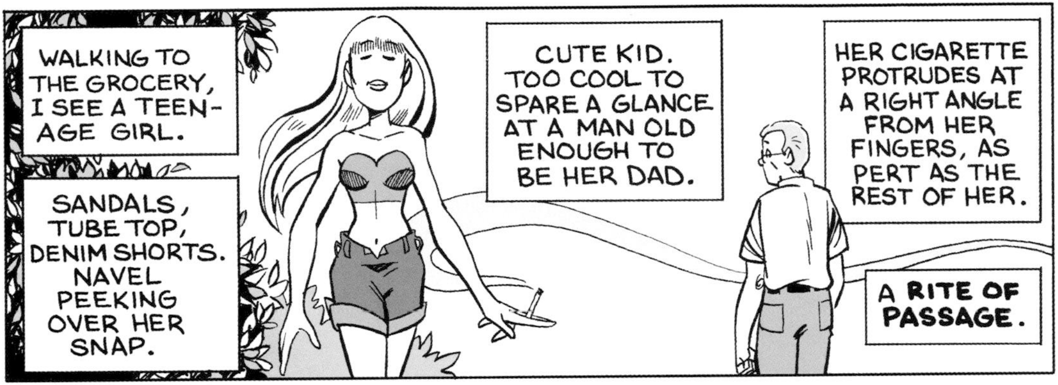
WALKING TO THE GROCERY, I SEE A TEEN-AGE GIRL.
SANDALS, TUBE TOP, DENIM SHORTS. NAVEL PEEKING OVER HER SNAP.
CUTE KID. TOO COOL TO SPARE A GLANCE AT A MAN OLD ENOUGH TO BE HER DAD.
HER CIGARETTE PROTRUDES AT A RIGHT ANGLE FROM HER FINGERS, AS PERT AS THE REST OF HER.
A RITE OF PASSAGE.

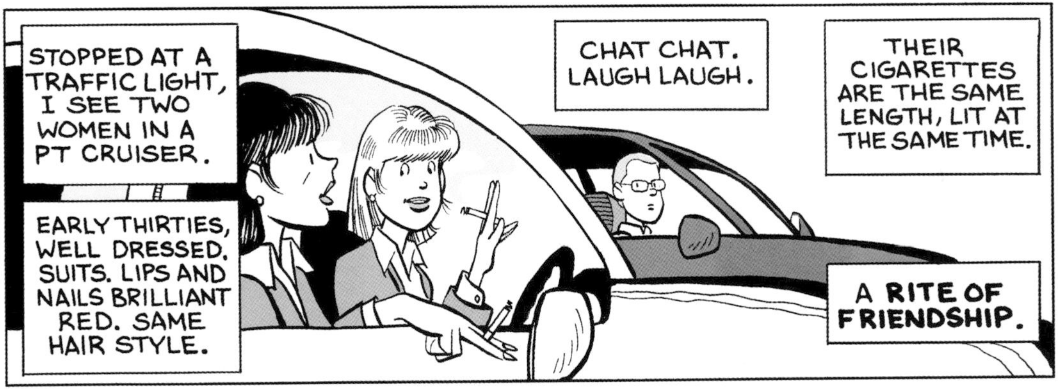
STOPPED AT A TRAFFIC LIGHT, I SEE TWO WOMEN IN A PT CRUISER.
EARLY THIRTIES, WELL DRESSED. SUITS. LIPS AND NAILS BRILLIANT RED. SAME HAIR STYLE.
CHAT CHAT. LAUGH LAUGH.
THEIR CIGARETTES ARE THE SAME LENGTH, LIT AT THE SAME TIME.
A RITE OF FRIENDSHIP.

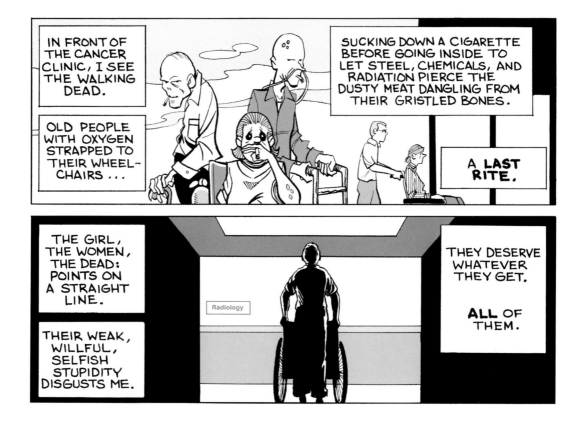

IN FRONT OF THE CANCER CLINIC, I SEE THE WALKING DEAD.

OLD PEOPLE WITH OXYGEN STRAPPED TO THEIR WHEEL-CHAIRS ...

SUCKING DOWN A CIGARETTE BEFORE GOING INSIDE TO LET STEEL, CHEMICALS, AND RADIATION PIERCE THE DUSTY MEAT DANGLING FROM THEIR GRISTLED BONES.

A **LAST** RITE.

THE GIRL, THE WOMEN, THE DEAD: POINTS ON A STRAIGHT LINE.

THEIR WEAK, WILLFUL, SELFISH STUPIDITY DISGUSTS ME.

Radiology

THEY DESERVE WHATEVER THEY GET.

ALL OF THEM.

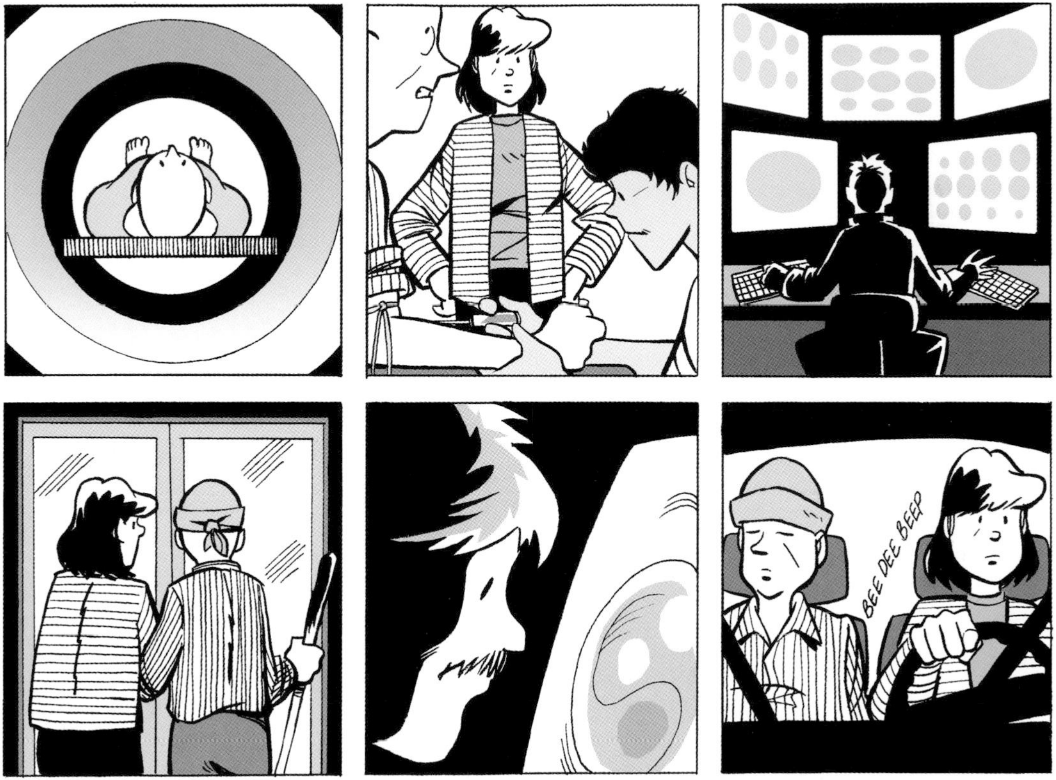
BEE DEE BEEP

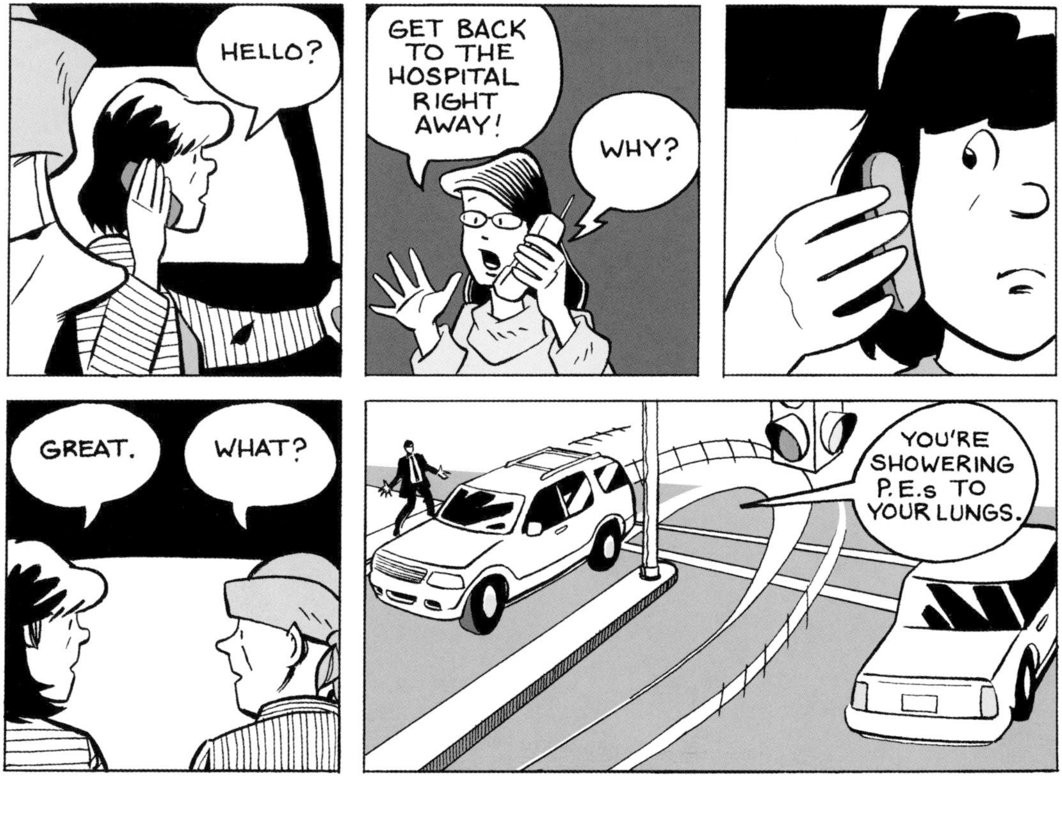
HELLO?
GET BACK TO THE HOSPITAL RIGHT AWAY!
WHY?
GREAT.
WHAT?
YOU'RE SHOWERING P.E.s TO YOUR LUNGS.

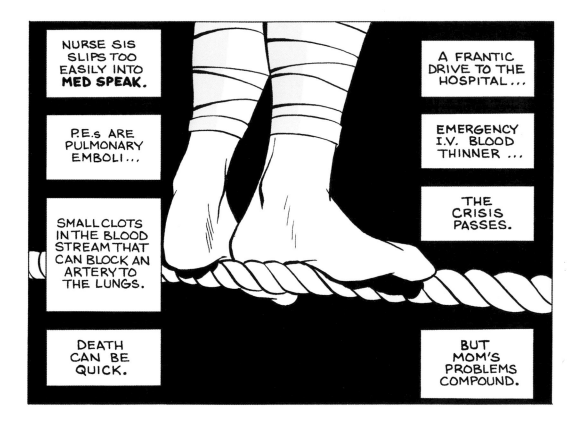

NURSE SIS SLIPS TOO EASILY INTO **MED SPEAK.**

P.E.s ARE PULMONARY EMBOLI...

SMALL CLOTS IN THE BLOOD STREAM THAT CAN BLOCK AN ARTERY TO THE LUNGS.

DEATH CAN BE QUICK.

A FRANTIC DRIVE TO THE HOSPITAL...

EMERGENCY I.V. BLOOD THINNER...

THE CRISIS PASSES.

BUT MOM'S PROBLEMS COMPOUND.

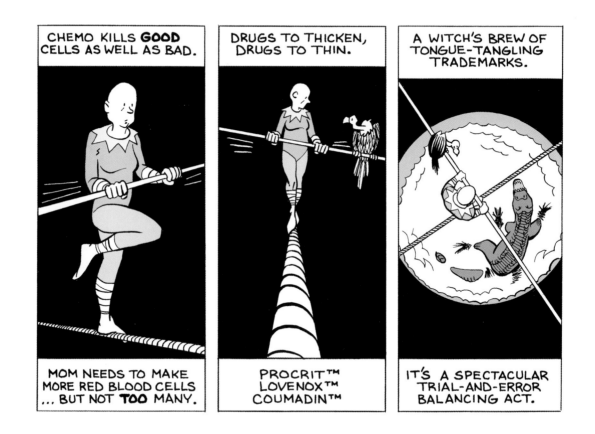

CHEMO KILLS **GOOD** CELLS AS WELL AS BAD.

MOM NEEDS TO MAKE MORE RED BLOOD CELLS ... BUT NOT **TOO** MANY.

DRUGS TO THICKEN, DRUGS TO THIN.

PROCRIT™ LOVENOX™ COUMADIN™

A WITCH'S BREW OF TONGUE-TANGLING TRADEMARKS.

IT'S A SPECTACULAR TRIAL-AND-ERROR BALANCING ACT.

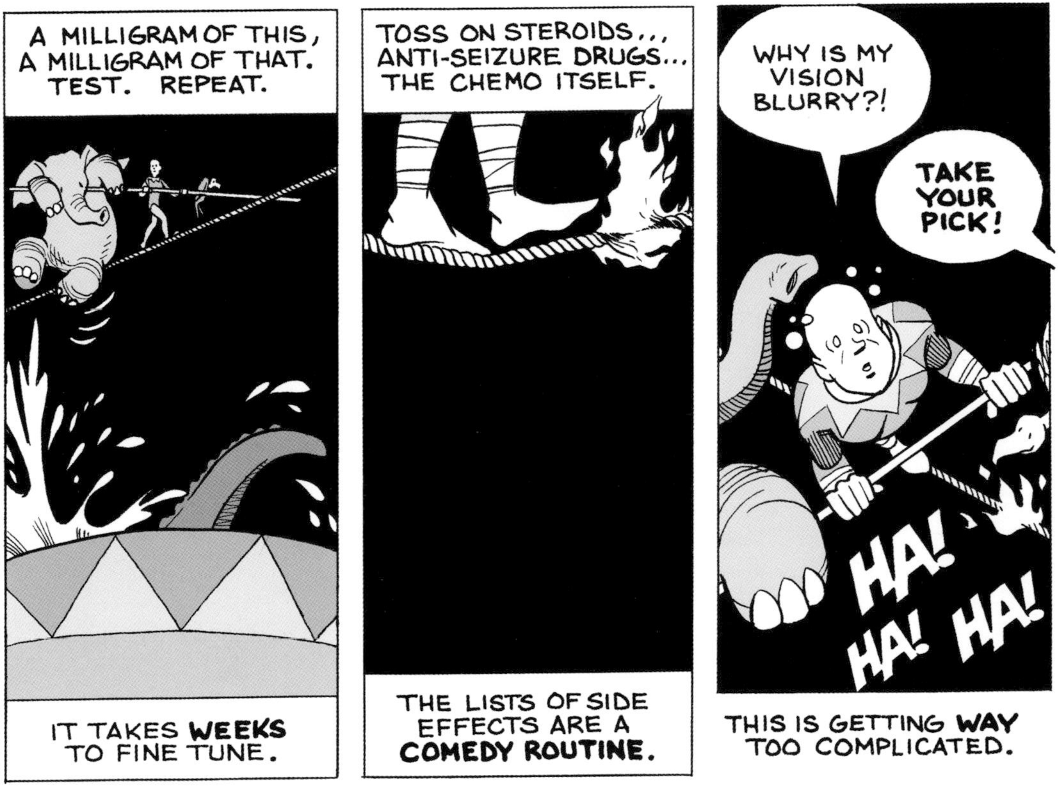
A MILLIGRAM OF THIS, A MILLIGRAM OF THAT. TEST. REPEAT.
IT TAKES **WEEKS** TO FINE TUNE.
TOSS ON STEROIDS... ANTI-SEIZURE DRUGS... THE CHEMO ITSELF.
THE LISTS OF SIDE EFFECTS ARE A **COMEDY ROUTINE**.
WHY IS MY VISION BLURRY?!
TAKE YOUR PICK!
HA! HA! HA!
THIS IS GETTING **WAY** TOO COMPLICATED.

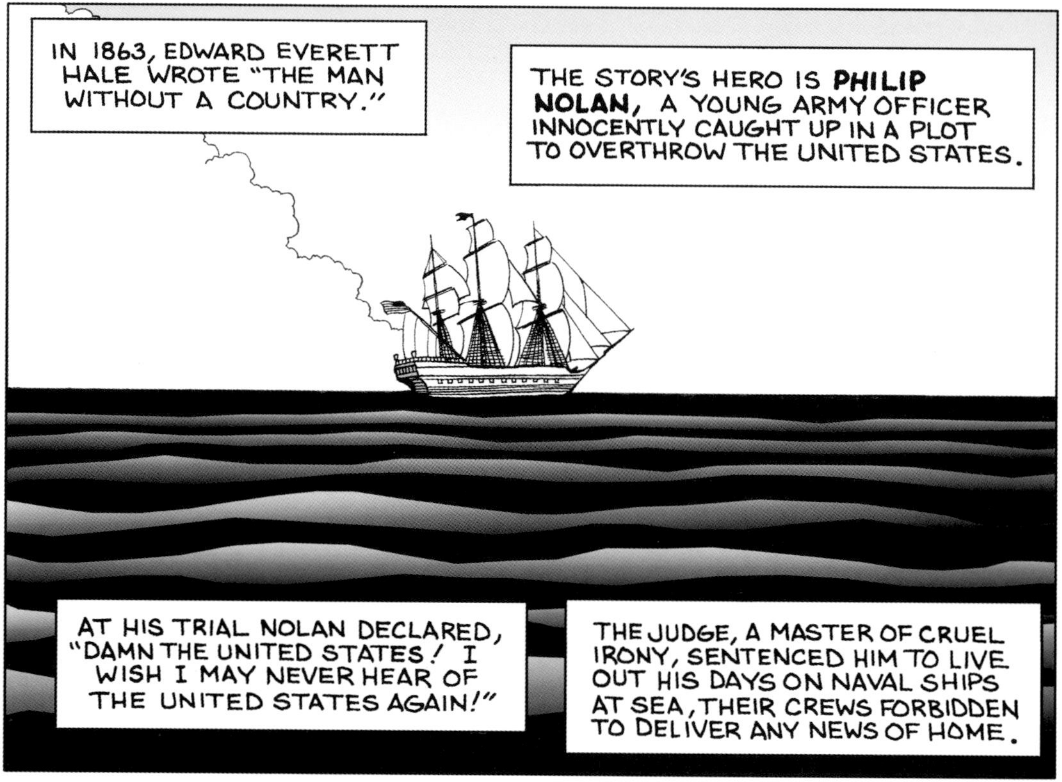
IN 1863, EDWARD EVERETT HALE WROTE "THE MAN WITHOUT A COUNTRY."
THE STORY'S HERO IS **PHILIP NOLAN**, A YOUNG ARMY OFFICER INNOCENTLY CAUGHT UP IN A PLOT TO OVERTHROW THE UNITED STATES.
AT HIS TRIAL NOLAN DECLARED, "DAMN THE UNITED STATES! I WISH I MAY NEVER HEAR OF THE UNITED STATES AGAIN!"
THE JUDGE, A MASTER OF CRUEL IRONY, SENTENCED HIM TO LIVE OUT HIS DAYS ON NAVAL SHIPS AT SEA, THEIR CREWS FORBIDDEN TO DELIVER ANY NEWS OF HOME.

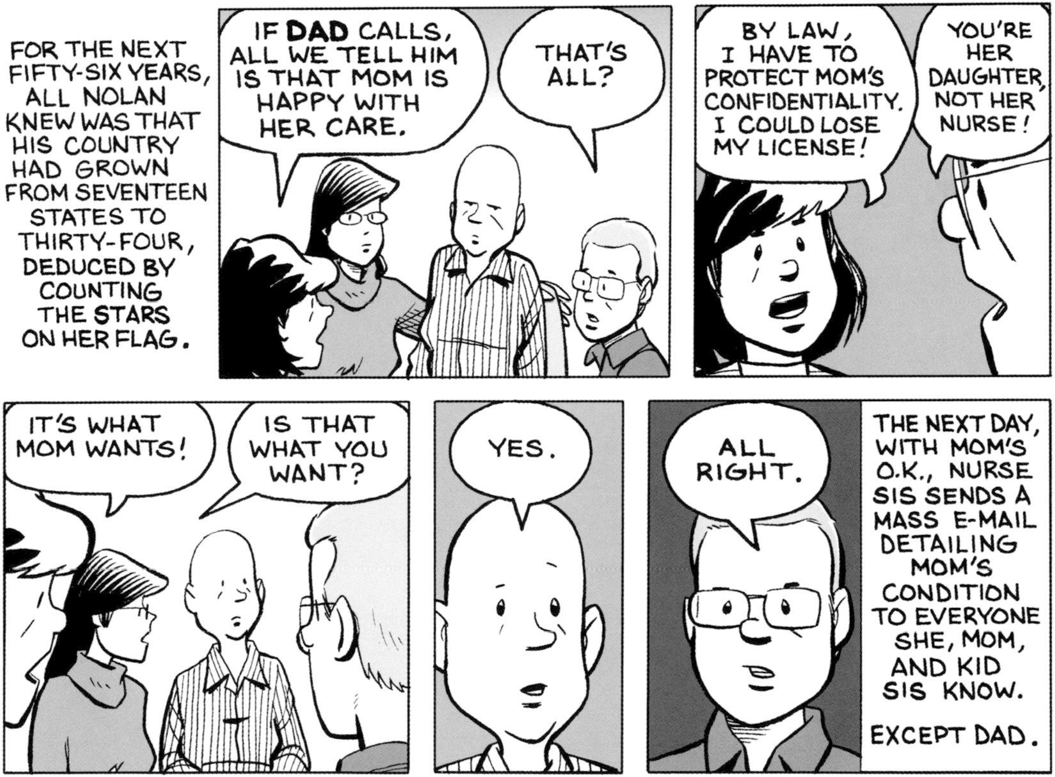

FOR THE NEXT FIFTY-SIX YEARS, ALL NOLAN KNEW WAS THAT HIS COUNTRY HAD GROWN FROM SEVENTEEN STATES TO THIRTY-FOUR, DEDUCED BY COUNTING THE STARS ON HER FLAG.
IF DAD CALLS, ALL WE TELL HIM IS THAT MOM IS HAPPY WITH HER CARE.
THAT'S ALL?
BY LAW, I HAVE TO PROTECT MOM'S CONFIDENTIALITY. I COULD LOSE MY LICENSE!
YOU'RE HER DAUGHTER, NOT HER NURSE!
IT'S WHAT MOM WANTS!
IS THAT WHAT YOU WANT?
YES.
ALL RIGHT.
THE NEXT DAY, WITH MOM'S O.K., NURSE SIS SENDS A MASS E-MAIL DETAILING MOM'S CONDITION TO EVERYONE SHE, MOM, AND KID SIS KNOW.
EXCEPT DAD.

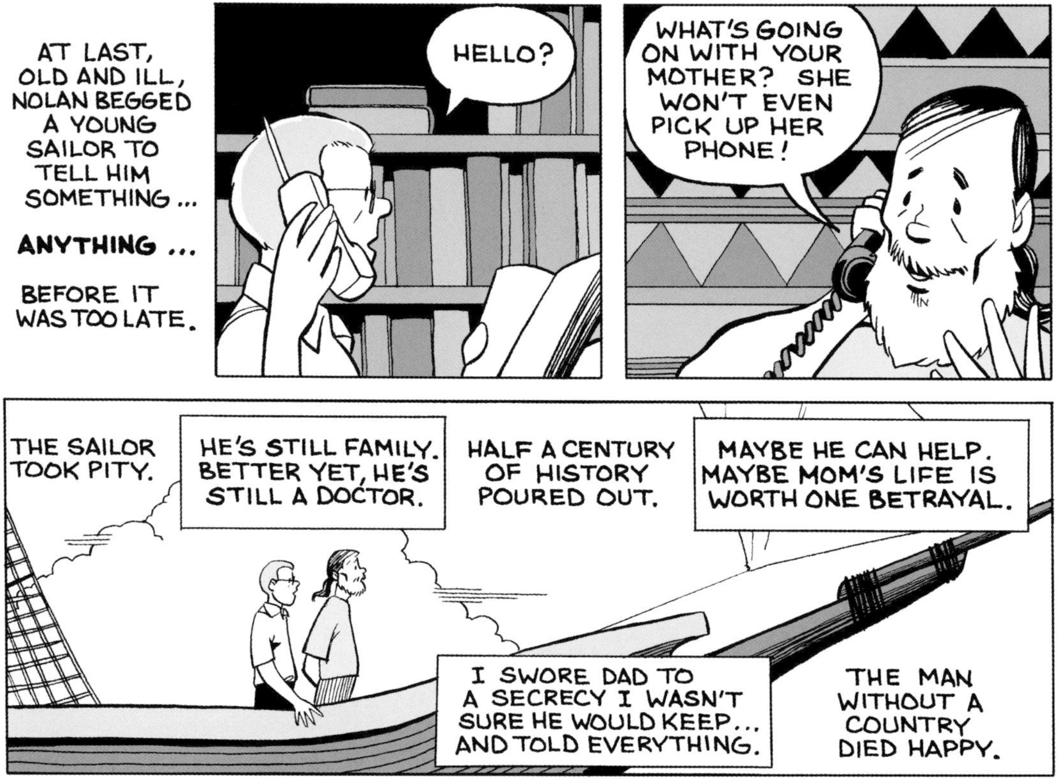
AT LAST, OLD AND ILL, NOLAN BEGGED A YOUNG SAILOR TO TELL HIM SOMETHING ...
ANYTHING ...
BEFORE IT WAS TOO LATE.
HELLO?
WHAT'S GOING ON WITH YOUR MOTHER? SHE WON'T EVEN PICK UP HER PHONE!
THE SAILOR TOOK PITY.
HE'S STILL FAMILY. BETTER YET, HE'S STILL A DOCTOR.
HALF A CENTURY OF HISTORY POURED OUT.
MAYBE HE CAN HELP. MAYBE MOM'S LIFE IS WORTH ONE BETRAYAL.
I SWORE DAD TO A SECRECY I WASN'T SURE HE WOULD KEEP... AND TOLD EVERYTHING.
THE MAN WITHOUT A COUNTRY DIED HAPPY.

THE NEXT DAY . . .

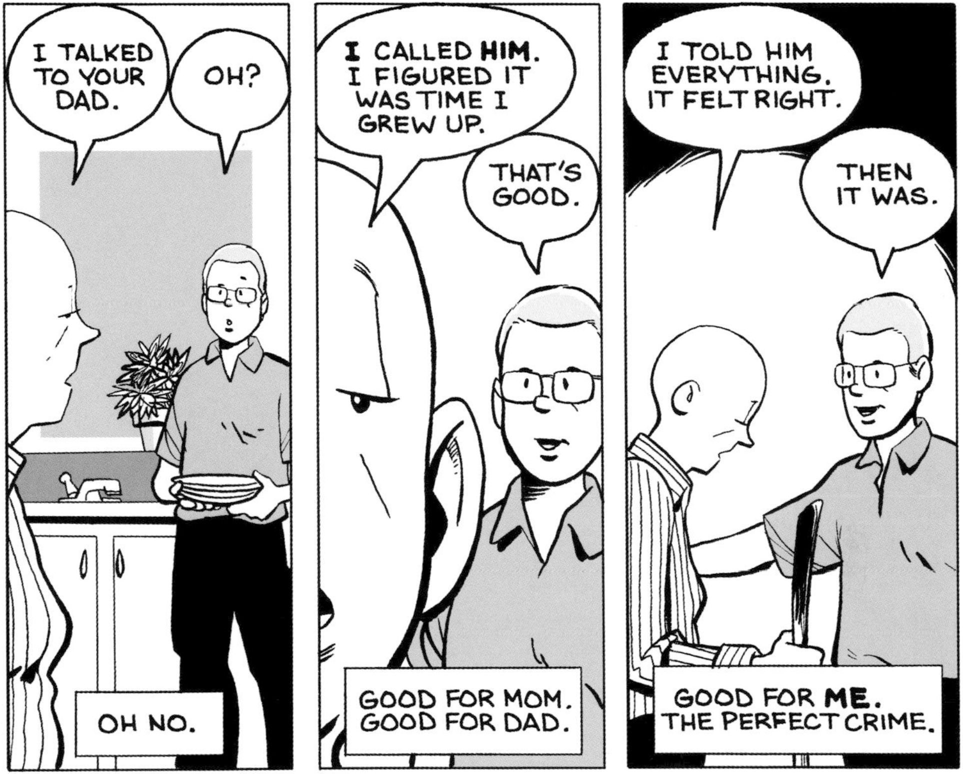
I TALKED TO YOUR DAD.
OH?
OH NO.
I CALLED HIM. I FIGURED IT WAS TIME I GREW UP.
THAT'S GOOD.
GOOD FOR MOM. GOOD FOR DAD.
I TOLD HIM EVERYTHING. IT FELT RIGHT.
THEN IT WAS.
GOOD FOR ME. THE PERFECT CRIME.

PUZZLEMENT

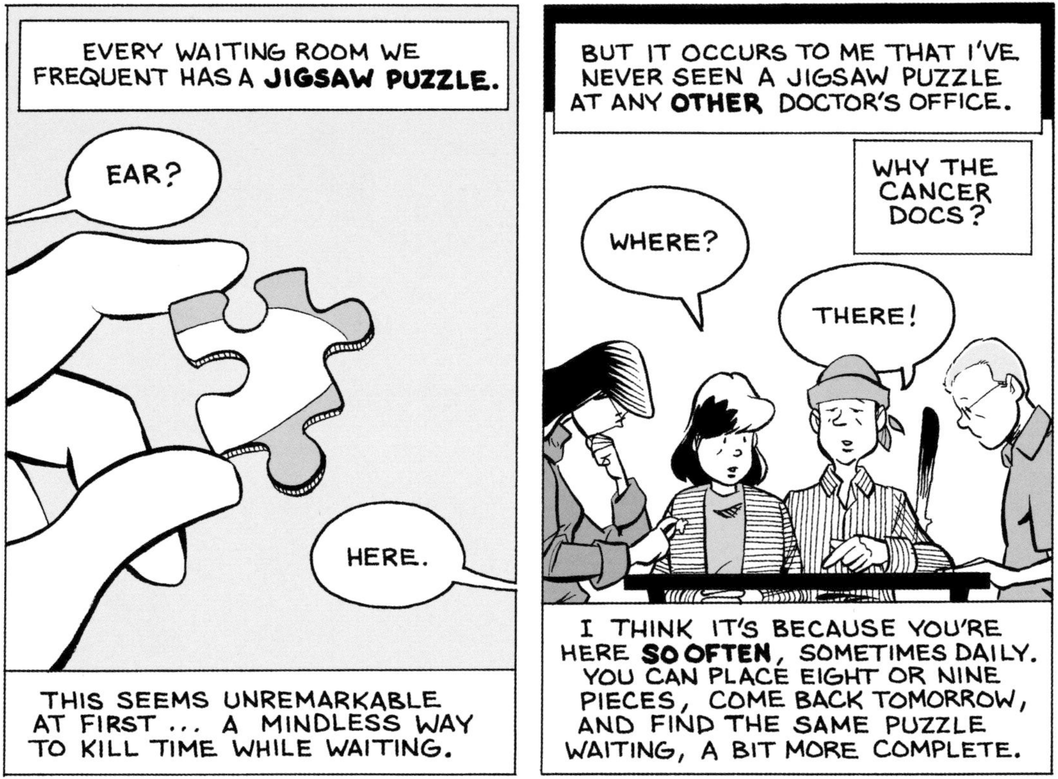
EVERY WAITING ROOM WE FREQUENT HAS A **JIGSAW PUZZLE.**
EAR?
HERE.
THIS SEEMS UNREMARKABLE AT FIRST ... A MINDLESS WAY TO KILL TIME WHILE WAITING.
BUT IT OCCURS TO ME THAT I'VE NEVER SEEN A JIGSAW PUZZLE AT ANY **OTHER** DOCTOR'S OFFICE.
WHY THE CANCER DOCS?
WHERE?
THERE!
I THINK IT'S BECAUSE YOU'RE HERE **SO OFTEN**, SOMETIMES DAILY. YOU CAN PLACE EIGHT OR NINE PIECES, COME BACK TOMORROW, AND FIND THE SAME PUZZLE WAITING, A BIT MORE COMPLETE.

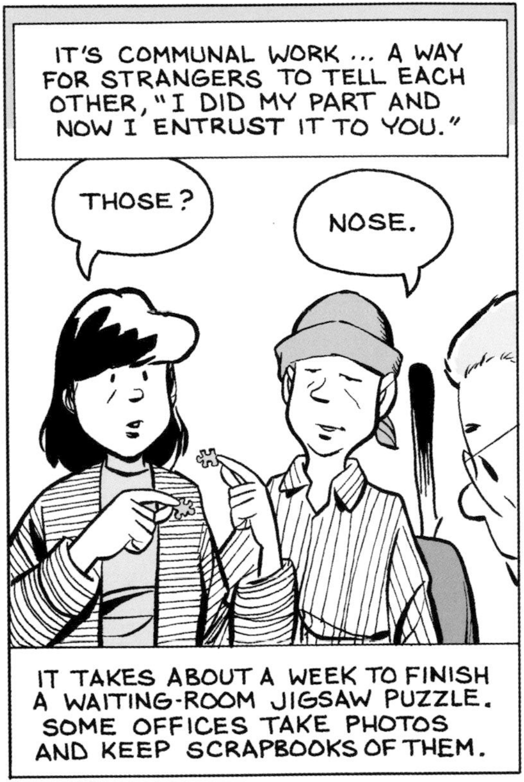
IT'S COMMUNAL WORK ... A WAY FOR STRANGERS TO TELL EACH OTHER, "I DID MY PART AND NOW I ENTRUST IT TO YOU."
THOSE?
NOSE.
IT TAKES ABOUT A WEEK TO FINISH A WAITING-ROOM JIGSAW PUZZLE. SOME OFFICES TAKE PHOTOS AND KEEP SCRAPBOOKS OF THEM.

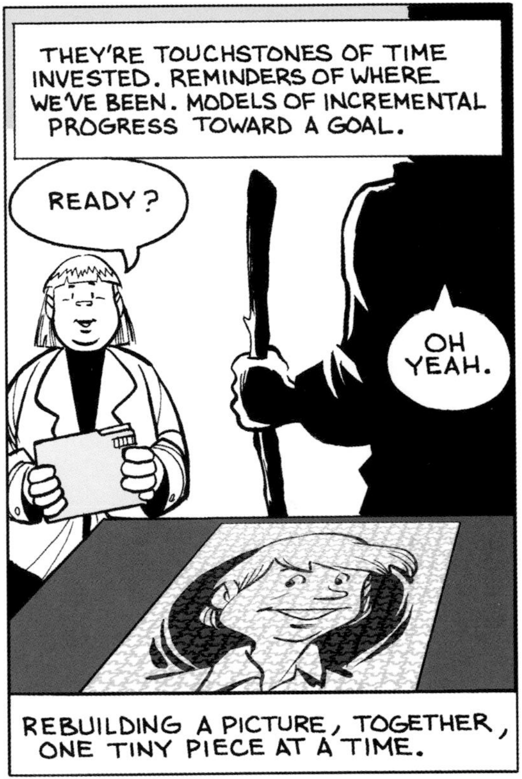
THEY'RE TOUCHSTONES OF TIME INVESTED. REMINDERS OF WHERE WE'VE BEEN. MODELS OF INCREMENTAL PROGRESS TOWARD A GOAL.
READY?
OH YEAH.
REBUILDING A PICTURE, TOGETHER, ONE TINY PIECE AT A TIME.

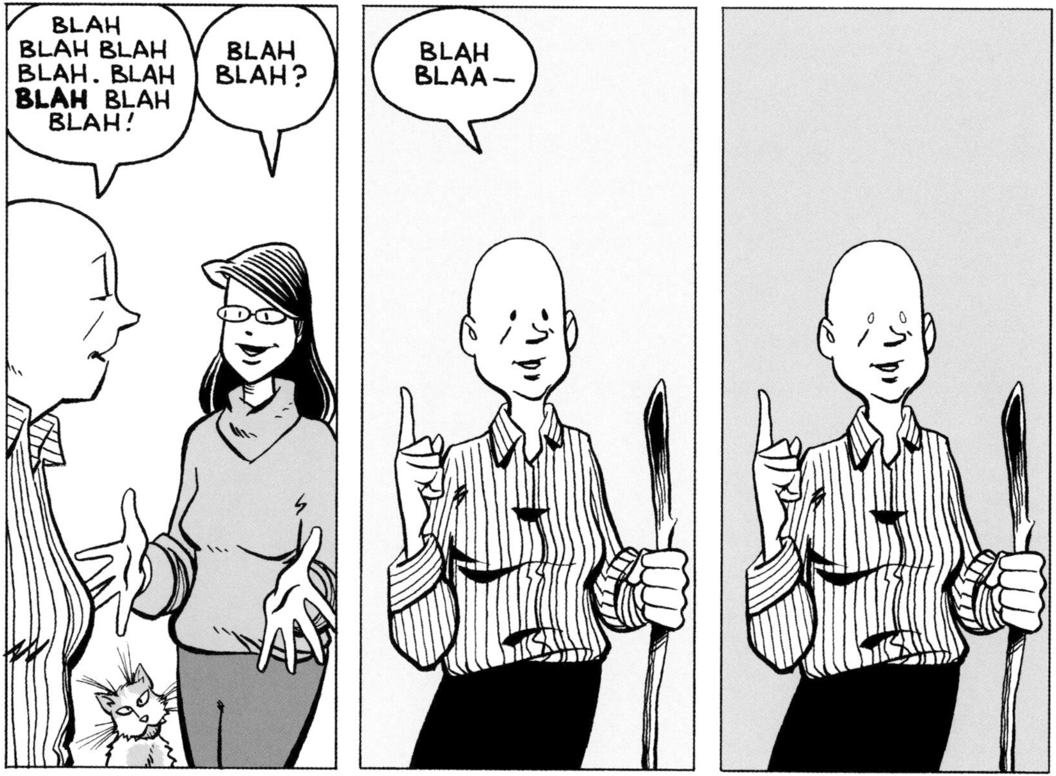
BLAH BLAH BLAH BLAH. BLAH **BLAH** BLAH BLAH!
BLAH BLAH?
BLAH BLAA—

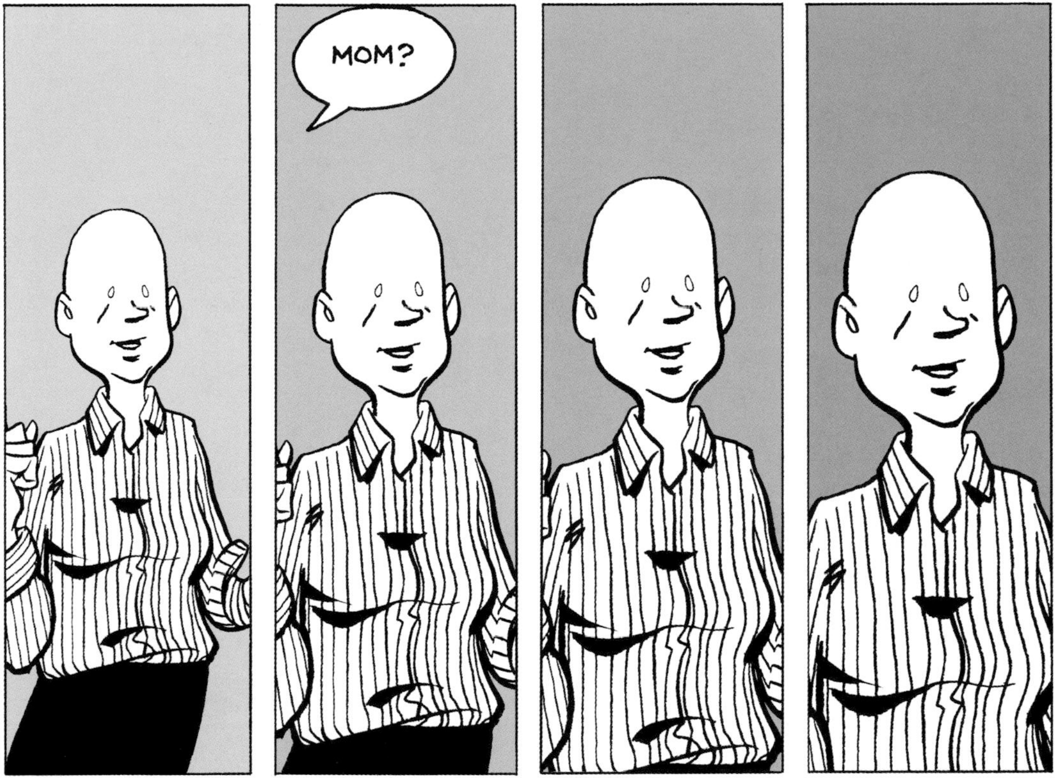
MOM?

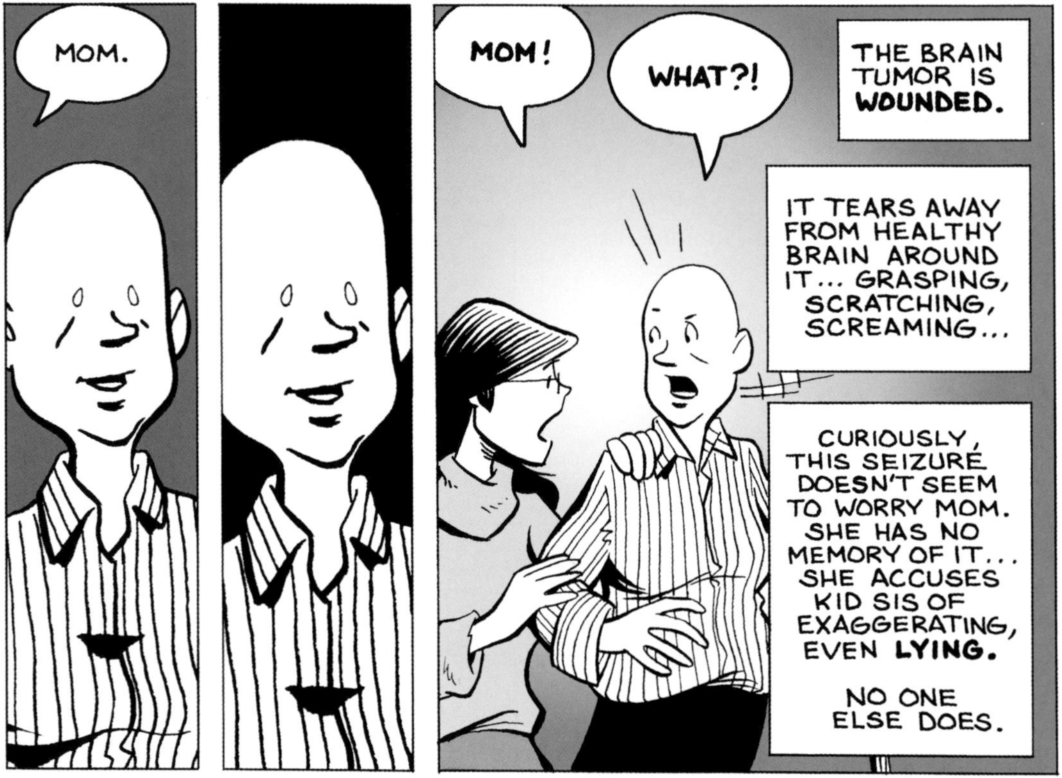
MOM.
MOM!
WHAT?!
THE BRAIN TUMOR IS WOUNDED.
IT TEARS AWAY FROM HEALTHY BRAIN AROUND IT... GRASPING, SCRATCHING, SCREAMING...
CURIOUSLY, THIS SEIZURE DOESN'T SEEM TO WORRY MOM. SHE HAS NO MEMORY OF IT... SHE ACCUSES KID SIS OF EXAGGERATING, EVEN LYING.
NO ONE ELSE DOES.

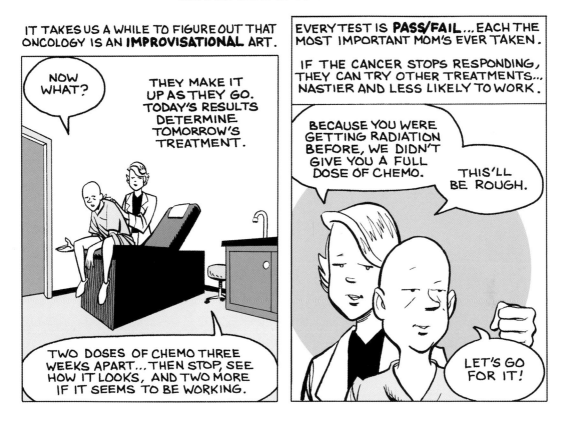

IT TAKES US A WHILE TO FIGURE OUT THAT ONCOLOGY IS AN **IMPROVISATIONAL** ART.

NOW WHAT?

THEY MAKE IT UP AS THEY GO. TODAY'S RESULTS DETERMINE TOMORROW'S TREATMENT.

TWO DOSES OF CHEMO THREE WEEKS APART... THEN STOP, SEE HOW IT LOOKS, AND TWO MORE IF IT SEEMS TO BE WORKING.

EVERY TEST IS **PASS/FAIL**... EACH THE MOST IMPORTANT MOM'S EVER TAKEN.

IF THE CANCER STOPS RESPONDING, THEY CAN TRY OTHER TREATMENTS... NASTIER AND LESS LIKELY TO WORK.

BECAUSE YOU WERE GETTING RADIATION BEFORE, WE DIDN'T GIVE YOU A FULL DOSE OF CHEMO.

THIS'LL BE ROUGH.

LET'S GO FOR IT!

71

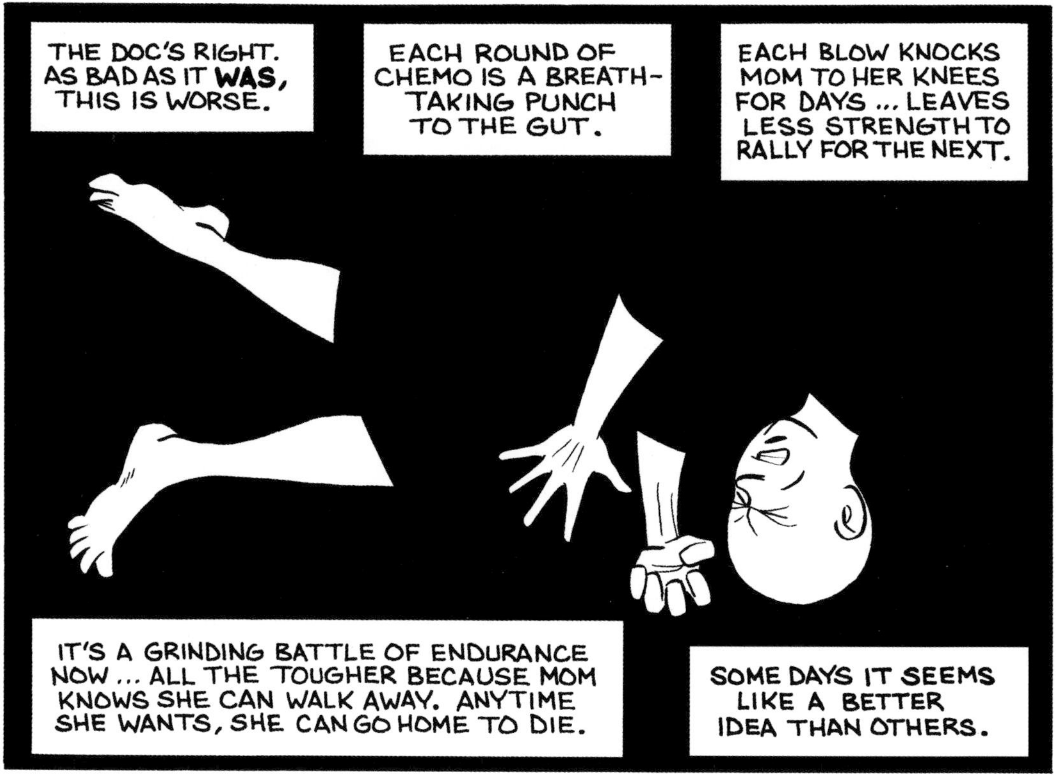
THE DOC'S RIGHT. AS BAD AS IT **WAS**, THIS IS WORSE.
EACH ROUND OF CHEMO IS A BREATH-TAKING PUNCH TO THE GUT.
EACH BLOW KNOCKS MOM TO HER KNEES FOR DAYS ... LEAVES LESS STRENGTH TO RALLY FOR THE NEXT.
IT'S A GRINDING BATTLE OF ENDURANCE NOW ... ALL THE TOUGHER BECAUSE MOM KNOWS SHE CAN WALK AWAY. ANYTIME SHE WANTS, SHE CAN GO HOME TO DIE.
SOME DAYS IT SEEMS LIKE A BETTER IDEA THAN OTHERS.

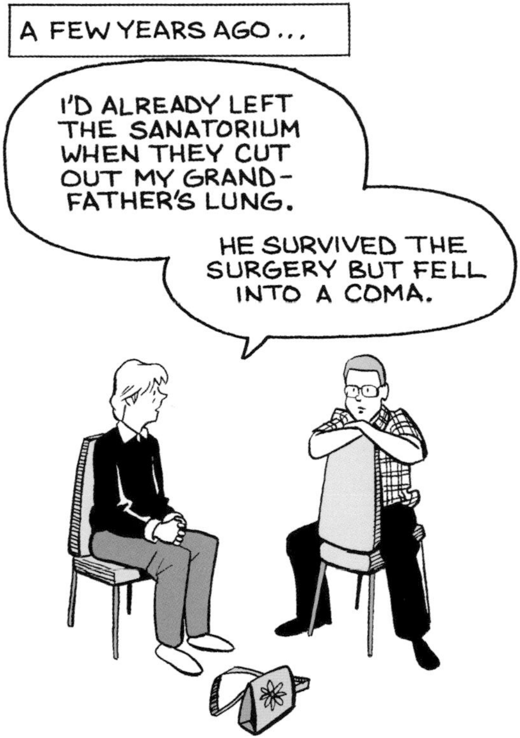
A FEW YEARS AGO...
I'D ALREADY LEFT THE SANATORIUM WHEN THEY CUT OUT MY GRAND-FATHER'S LUNG.
HE SURVIVED THE SURGERY BUT FELL INTO A COMA.

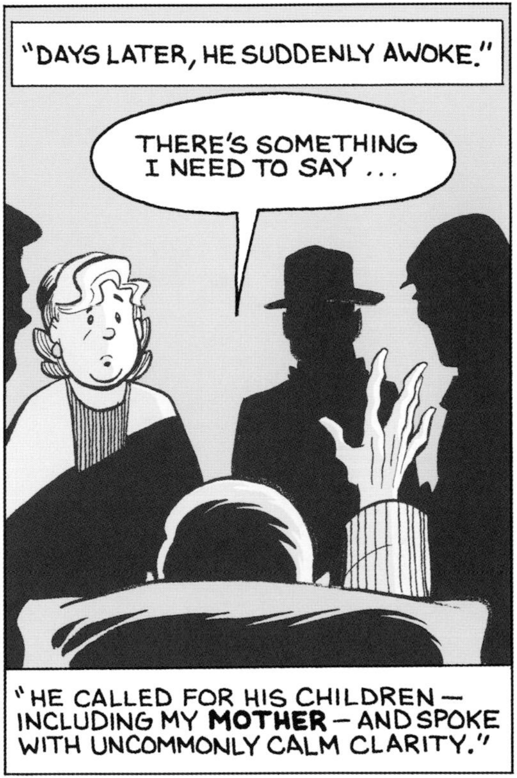
"DAYS LATER, HE SUDDENLY AWOKE."
THERE'S SOMETHING I NEED TO SAY ...
"HE CALLED FOR HIS CHILDREN — INCLUDING MY **MOTHER** — AND SPOKE WITH UNCOMMONLY CALM CLARITY."

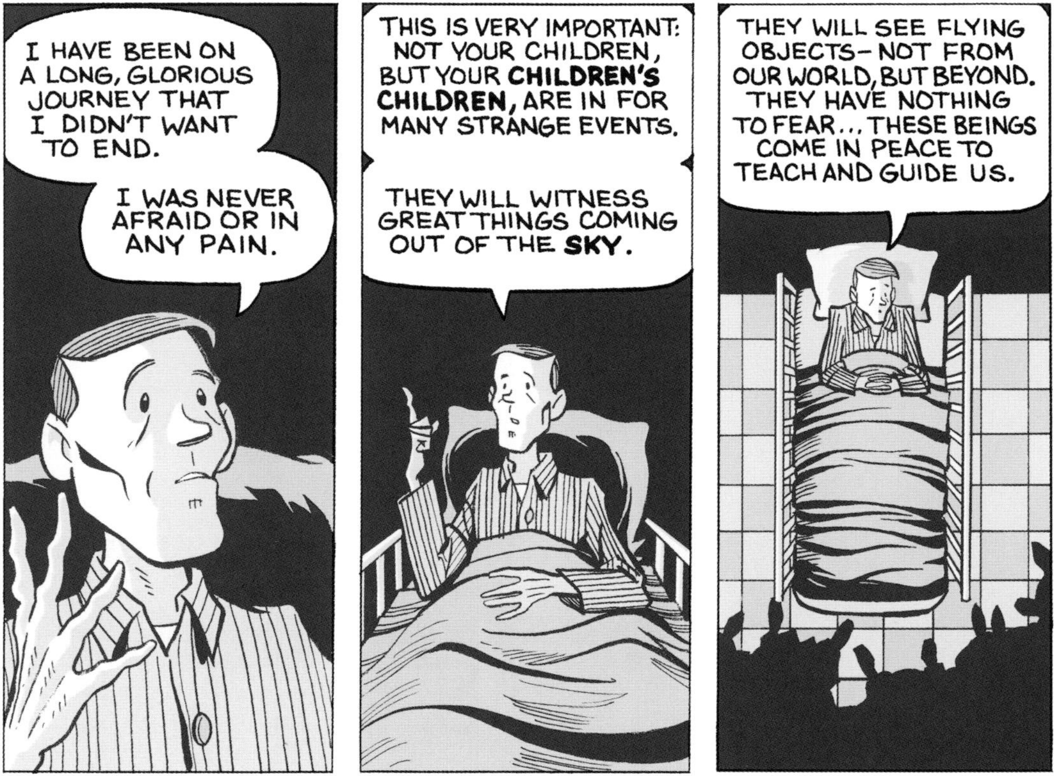
I HAVE BEEN ON A LONG, GLORIOUS JOURNEY THAT I DIDN'T WANT TO END.
I WAS NEVER AFRAID OR IN ANY PAIN.
THIS IS VERY IMPORTANT: NOT YOUR CHILDREN, BUT YOUR **CHILDREN'S CHILDREN**, ARE IN FOR MANY STRANGE EVENTS.
THEY WILL WITNESS GREAT THINGS COMING OUT OF THE **SKY**.
THEY WILL SEE FLYING OBJECTS— NOT FROM OUR WORLD, BUT BEYOND. THEY HAVE NOTHING TO FEAR... THESE BEINGS COME IN PEACE TO TEACH AND GUIDE US.

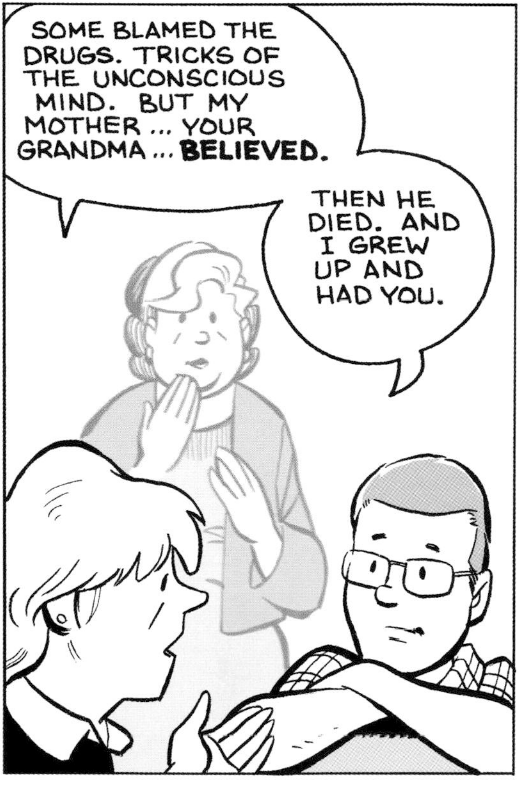
SOME BLAMED THE DRUGS. TRICKS OF THE UNCONSCIOUS MIND. BUT MY MOTHER ... YOUR GRANDMA ... **BELIEVED.**
THEN HE DIED. AND I GREW UP AND HAD YOU.

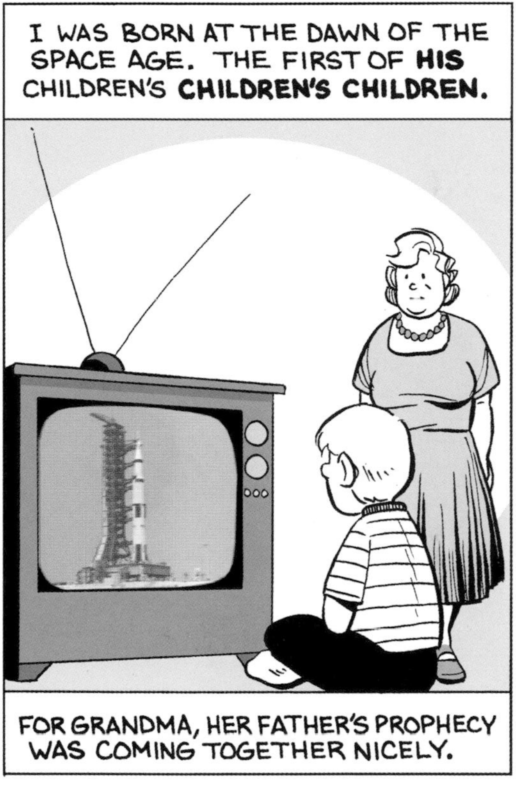
I WAS BORN AT THE DAWN OF THE SPACE AGE. THE FIRST OF **HIS** CHILDREN'S **CHILDREN'S CHILDREN.**
FOR GRANDMA, HER FATHER'S PROPHECY WAS COMING TOGETHER NICELY.

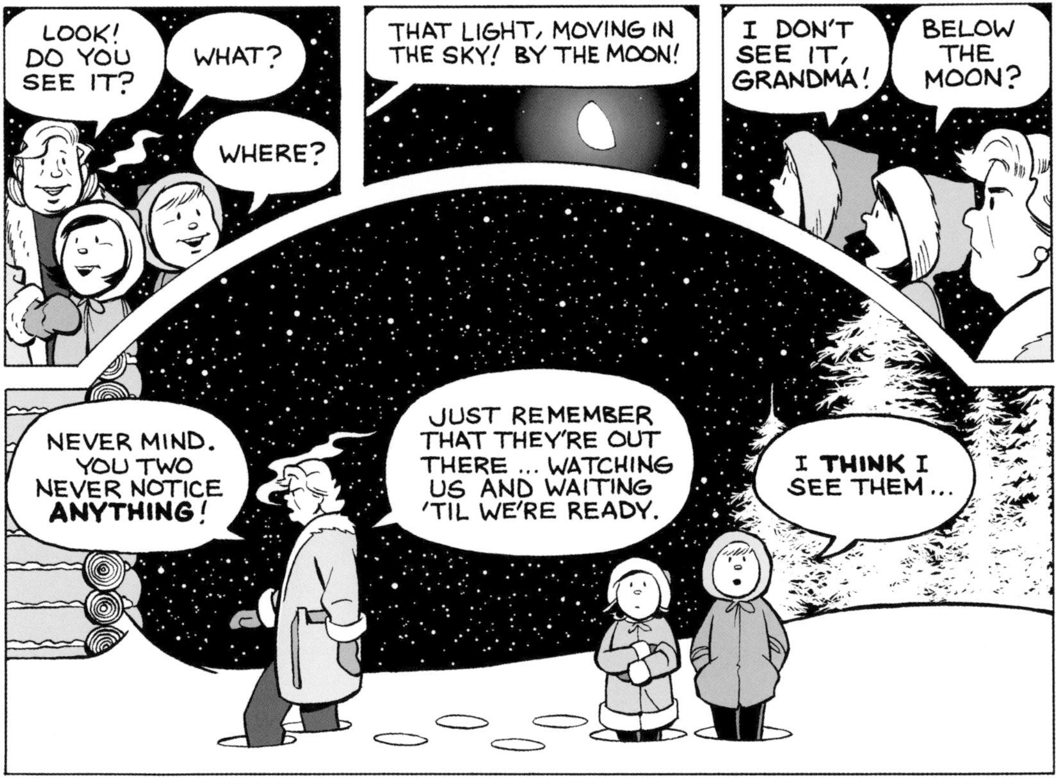
LOOK! DO YOU SEE IT?
WHAT?
WHERE?
THAT LIGHT, MOVING IN THE SKY! BY THE MOON!
I DON'T SEE IT, GRANDMA!
BELOW THE MOON?
NEVER MIND. YOU TWO NEVER NOTICE **ANYTHING**!
JUST REMEMBER THAT THEY'RE OUT THERE ... WATCHING US AND WAITING 'TIL WE'RE READY.
I **THINK** I SEE THEM ...

76

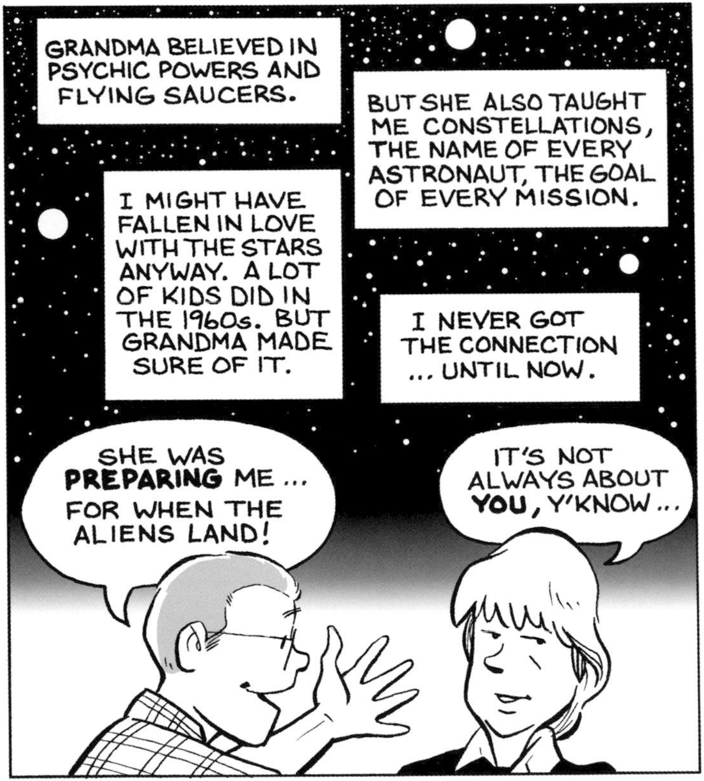
GRANDMA BELIEVED IN PSYCHIC POWERS AND FLYING SAUCERS.
BUT SHE ALSO TAUGHT ME CONSTELLATIONS, THE NAME OF EVERY ASTRONAUT, THE GOAL OF EVERY MISSION.
I MIGHT HAVE FALLEN IN LOVE WITH THE STARS ANYWAY. A LOT OF KIDS DID IN THE 1960s. BUT GRANDMA MADE SURE OF IT.
I NEVER GOT THE CONNECTION ... UNTIL NOW.
SHE WAS **PREPARING** ME ... FOR WHEN THE ALIENS LAND!
IT'S NOT ALWAYS ABOUT **YOU**, Y'KNOW ...

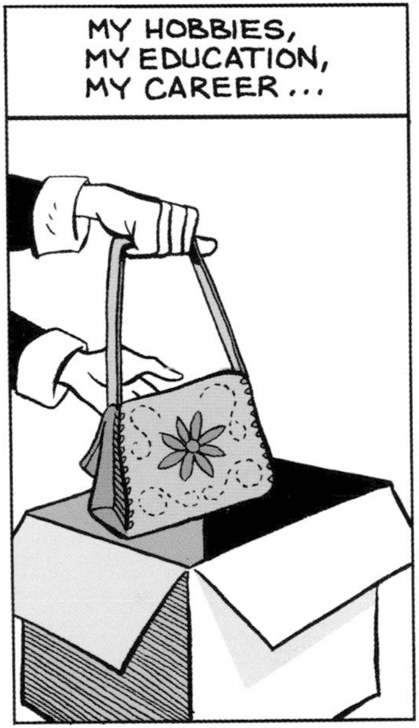
MY HOBBIES, MY EDUCATION, MY CAREER ...

DOES MY ENTIRE LIFE HINGE ON THE VISION OF A MAN WHO DIED YEARS BEFORE MY BIRTH?

IF SO, I OWE HIM ONE.

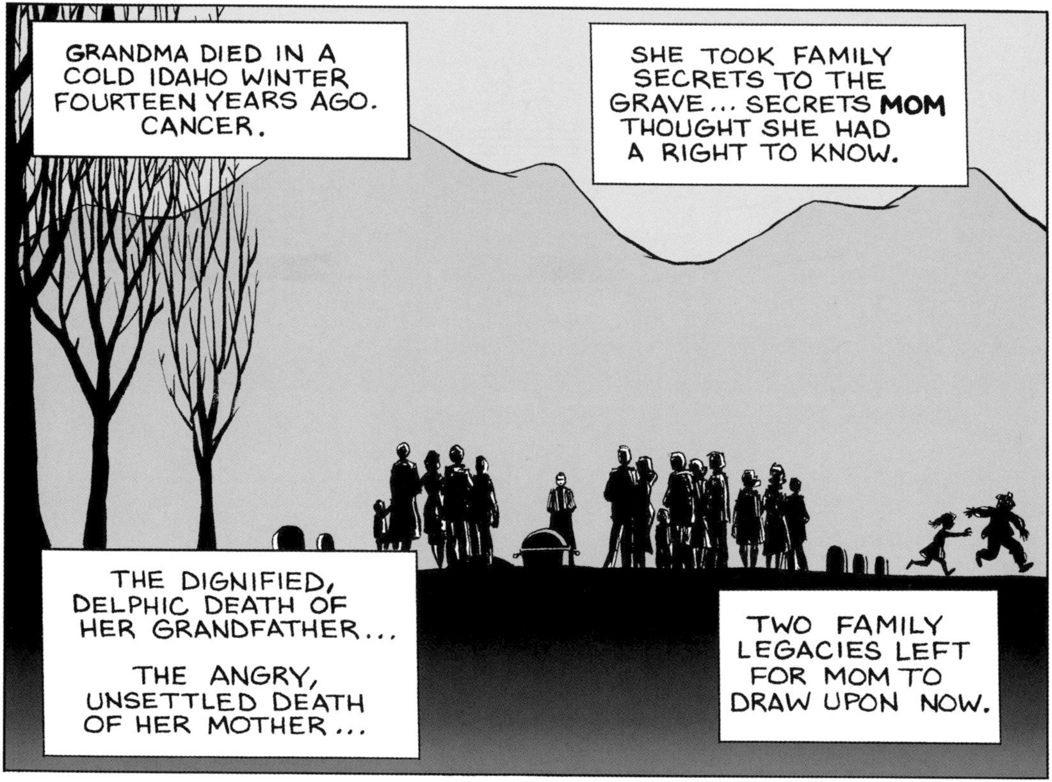
GRANDMA DIED IN A COLD IDAHO WINTER FOURTEEN YEARS AGO. CANCER.
SHE TOOK FAMILY SECRETS TO THE GRAVE... SECRETS **MOM** THOUGHT SHE HAD A RIGHT TO KNOW.
THE DIGNIFIED, DELPHIC DEATH OF HER GRANDFATHER...
THE ANGRY, UNSETTLED DEATH OF HER MOTHER...
TWO FAMILY LEGACIES LEFT FOR MOM TO DRAW UPON NOW.

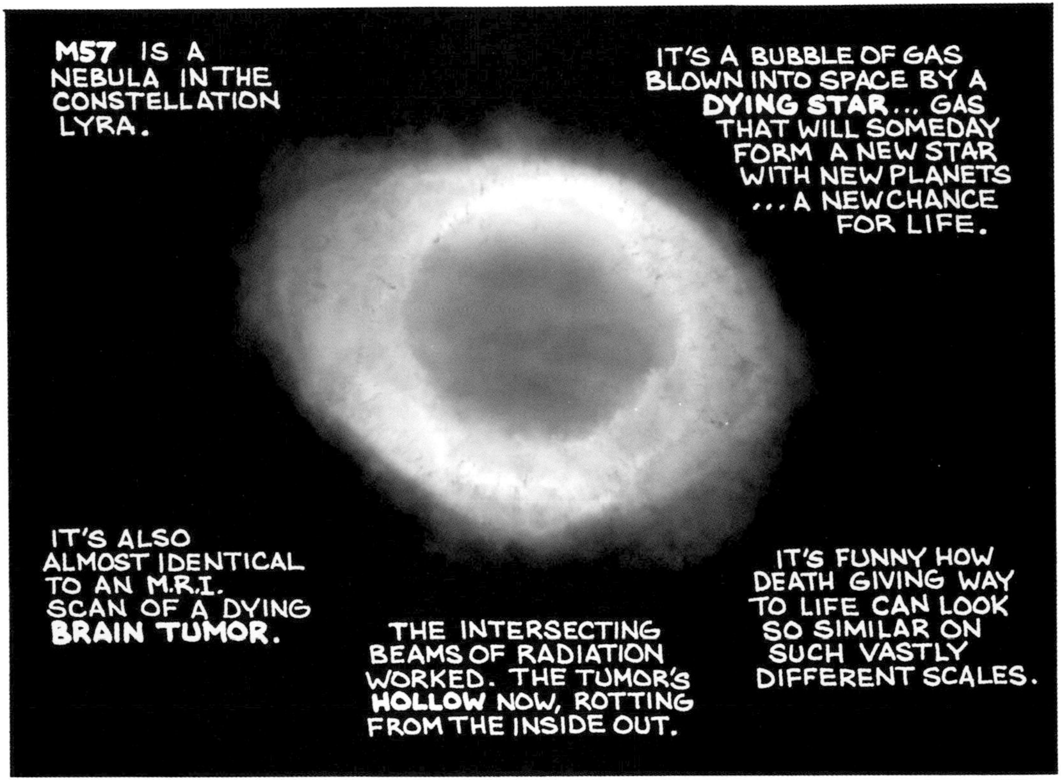
M57 IS A NEBULA IN THE CONSTELLATION LYRA.
IT'S A BUBBLE OF GAS BLOWN INTO SPACE BY A DYING STAR... GAS THAT WILL SOMEDAY FORM A NEW STAR WITH NEW PLANETS ... A NEW CHANCE FOR LIFE.
IT'S ALSO ALMOST IDENTICAL TO AN M.R.I. SCAN OF A DYING BRAIN TUMOR.
THE INTERSECTING BEAMS OF RADIATION WORKED. THE TUMOR'S HOLLOW NOW, ROTTING FROM THE INSIDE OUT.
IT'S FUNNY HOW DEATH GIVING WAY TO LIFE CAN LOOK SO SIMILAR ON SUCH VASTLY DIFFERENT SCALES.

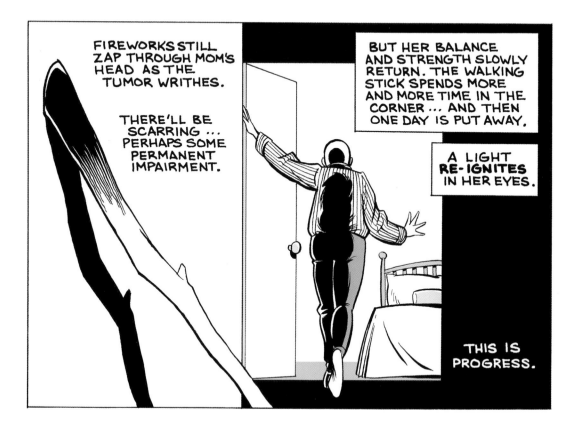

FIREWORKS STILL ZAP THROUGH MOM'S HEAD AS THE TUMOR WRITHES.

THERE'LL BE SCARRING ... PERHAPS SOME PERMANENT IMPAIRMENT.

BUT HER BALANCE AND STRENGTH SLOWLY RETURN. THE WALKING STICK SPENDS MORE AND MORE TIME IN THE CORNER ... AND THEN ONE DAY IS PUT AWAY.

A LIGHT **RE-IGNITES** IN HER EYES.

THIS IS PROGRESS.

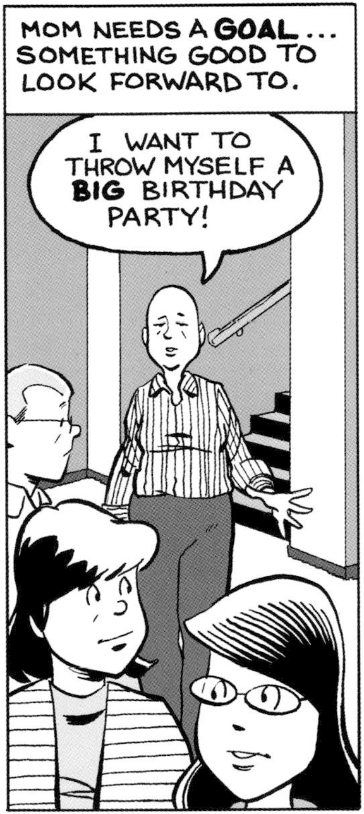
MOM NEEDS A **GOAL**... SOMETHING GOOD TO LOOK FORWARD TO.
I WANT TO THROW MYSELF A **BIG** BIRTHDAY PARTY!

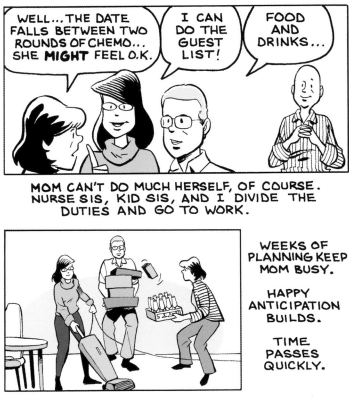

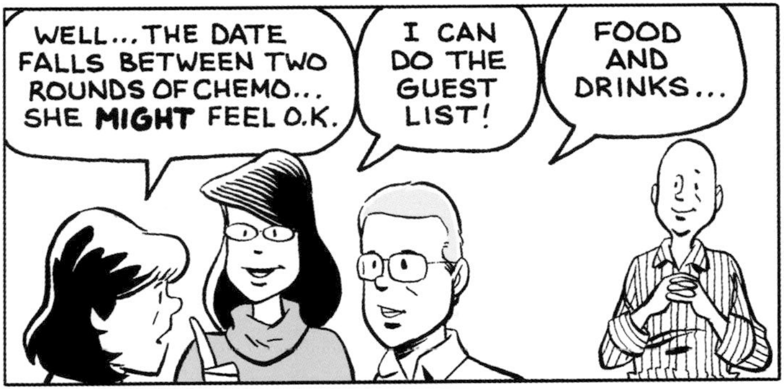
WELL... THE DATE FALLS BETWEEN TWO ROUNDS OF CHEMO... SHE **MIGHT** FEEL O.K.
I CAN DO THE GUEST LIST!
FOOD AND DRINKS...

MOM CAN'T DO MUCH HERSELF, OF COURSE. NURSE SIS, KID SIS, AND I DIVIDE THE DUTIES AND GO TO WORK.

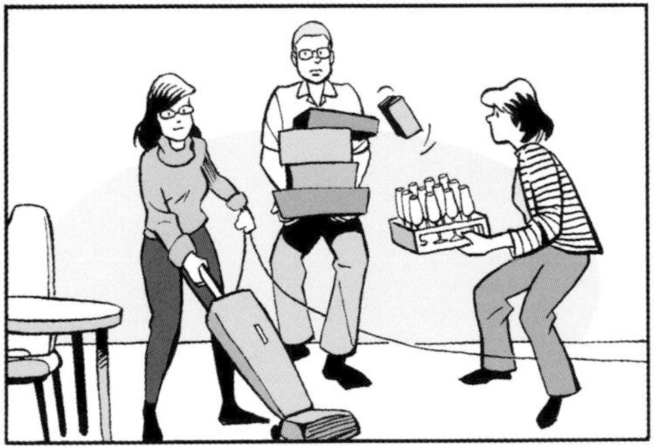

WEEKS OF PLANNING KEEP MOM BUSY.

HAPPY ANTICIPATION BUILDS.

TIME PASSES QUICKLY.

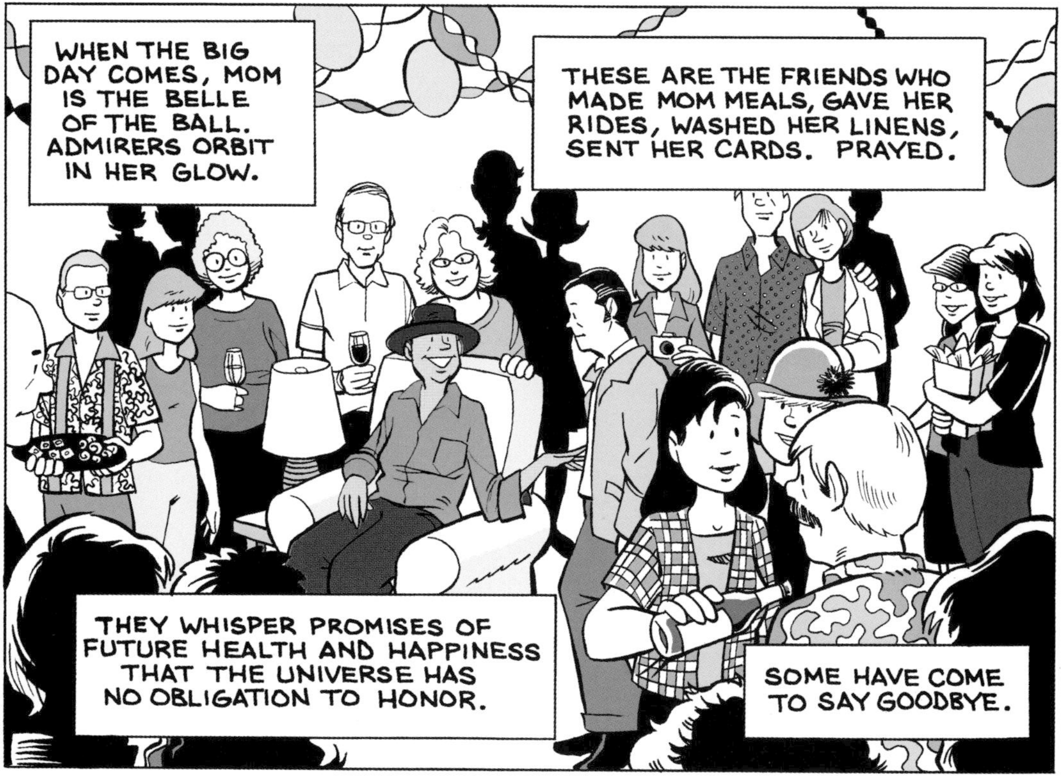
WHEN THE BIG DAY COMES, MOM IS THE BELLE OF THE BALL. ADMIRERS ORBIT IN HER GLOW.
THESE ARE THE FRIENDS WHO MADE MOM MEALS, GAVE HER RIDES, WASHED HER LINENS, SENT HER CARDS. PRAYED.
THEY WHISPER PROMISES OF FUTURE HEALTH AND HAPPINESS THAT THE UNIVERSE HAS NO OBLIGATION TO HONOR.
SOME HAVE COME TO SAY GOODBYE.

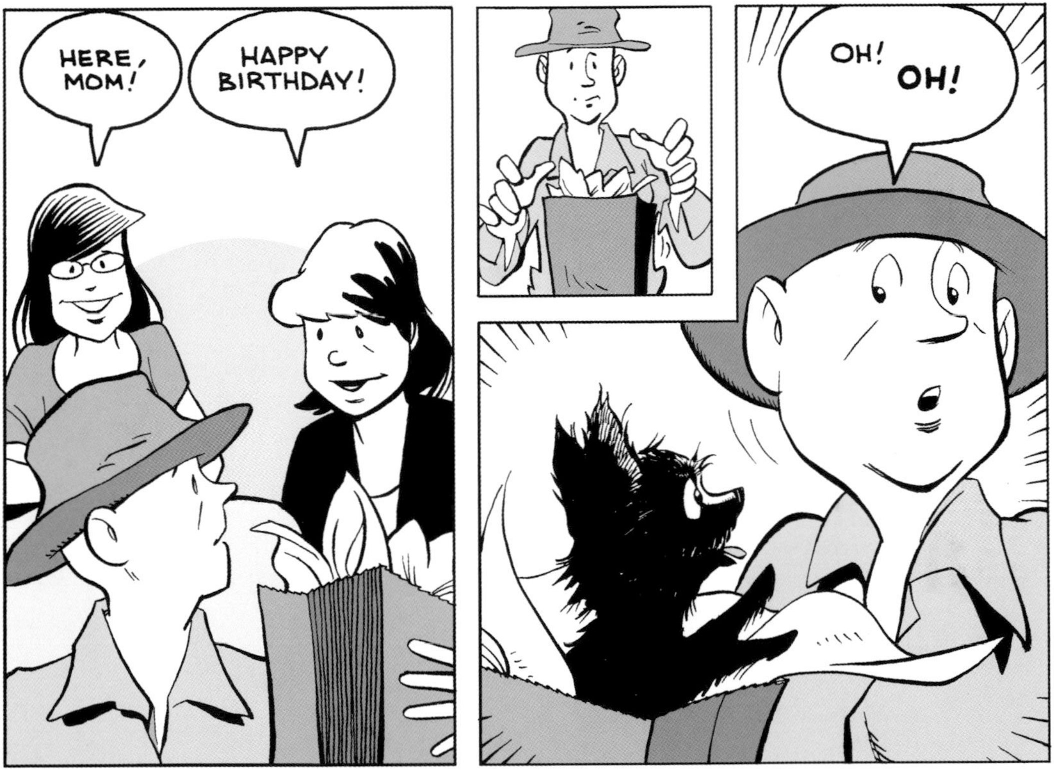
HERE, MOM!
HAPPY BIRTHDAY!
OH! OH!

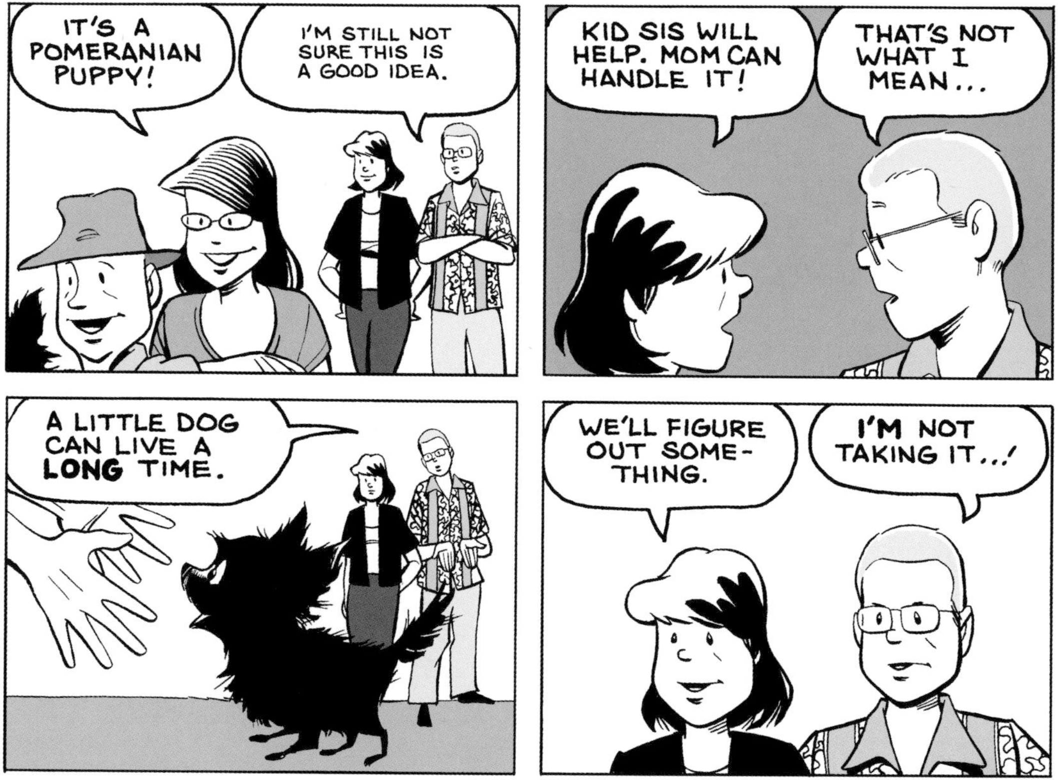
IT'S A POMERANIAN PUPPY!
I'M STILL NOT SURE THIS IS A GOOD IDEA.
KID SIS WILL HELP. MOM CAN HANDLE IT!
THAT'S NOT WHAT I MEAN...
A LITTLE DOG CAN LIVE A **LONG** TIME.
WE'LL FIGURE OUT SOME-THING.
I'M NOT TAKING IT...!

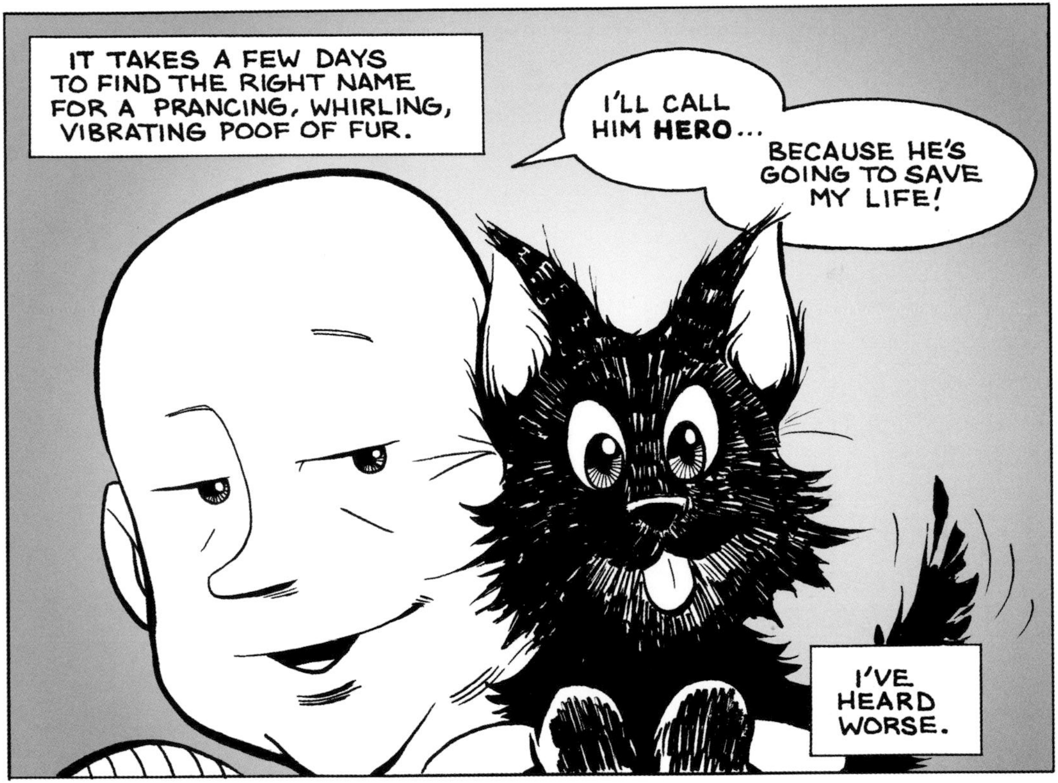
IT TAKES A FEW DAYS TO FIND THE RIGHT NAME FOR A PRANCING, WHIRLING, VIBRATING POOF OF FUR.
I'LL CALL HIM **HERO**...
BECAUSE HE'S GOING TO SAVE MY LIFE!
I'VE HEARD WORSE.

EVERY IMPORTANT CONVERSATION HAS **TWO** PARTS:

THE **TEXT** OF WORDS SPOKEN...

AND THE UNSPOKEN **SUBTEXT** OF WHAT THOSE WORDS REALLY MEAN.

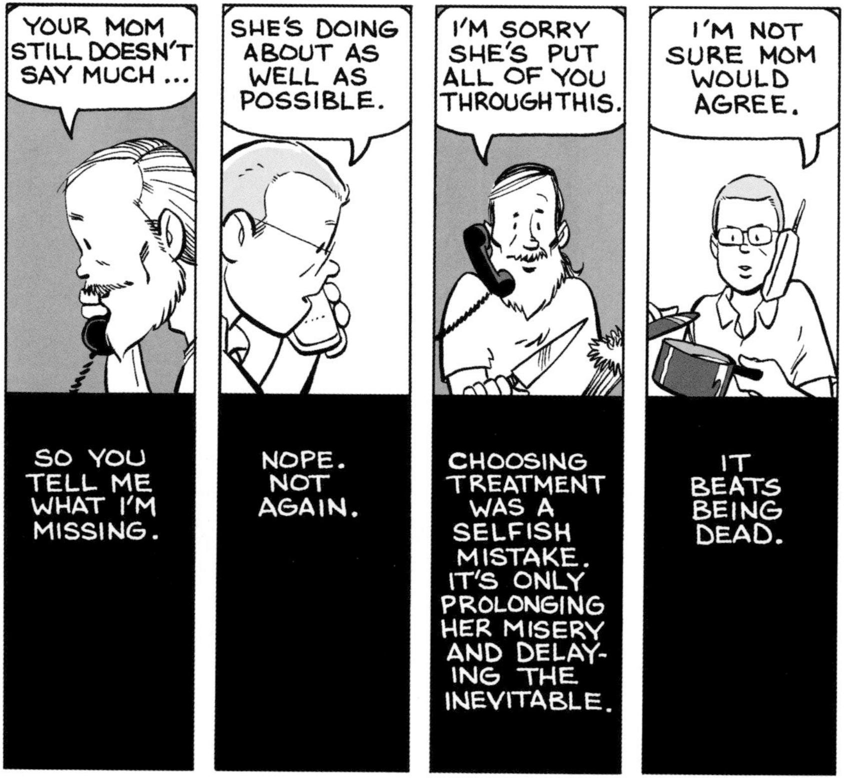
YOUR MOM STILL DOESN'T SAY MUCH...
SO YOU TELL ME WHAT I'M MISSING.
SHE'S DOING ABOUT AS WELL AS POSSIBLE.
NOPE. NOT AGAIN.
I'M SORRY SHE'S PUT ALL OF YOU THROUGH THIS.
CHOOSING TREATMENT WAS A SELFISH MISTAKE. IT'S ONLY PROLONGING HER MISERY AND DELAYING THE INEVITABLE.
I'M NOT SURE MOM WOULD AGREE.
IT BEATS BEING DEAD.

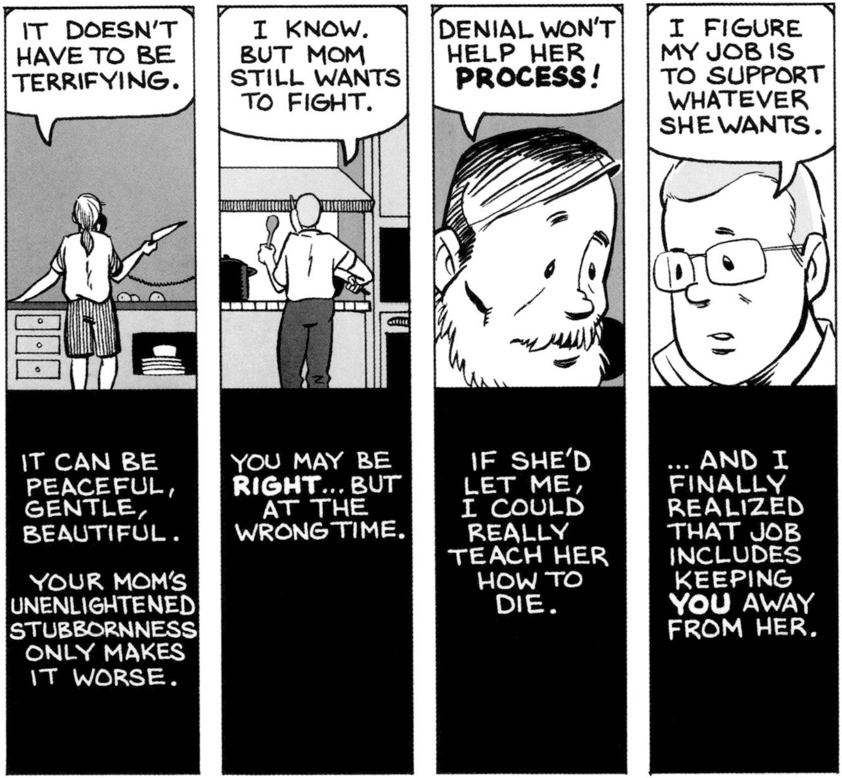
IT DOESN'T HAVE TO BE TERRIFYING.
IT CAN BE PEACEFUL, GENTLE, BEAUTIFUL.
YOUR MOM'S UNENLIGHTENED STUBBORNNESS ONLY MAKES IT WORSE.
I KNOW. BUT MOM STILL WANTS TO FIGHT.
YOU MAY BE **RIGHT**... BUT AT THE WRONG TIME.
DENIAL WON'T HELP HER **PROCESS**!
IF SHE'D LET ME, I COULD REALLY TEACH HER HOW TO DIE.
I FIGURE MY JOB IS TO SUPPORT WHATEVER SHE WANTS.
... AND I FINALLY REALIZED THAT JOB INCLUDES KEEPING **YOU** AWAY FROM HER.

GOODBYE.

WHEN DID WE ALL GET SO **CHUMMY** WITH DEATH?

EVERYBODY KNOWS THE **FIVE STAGES** OF GRIEF:

DENIAL, ANGER, BARGAINING, DEPRESSION, ACCEPTANCE.

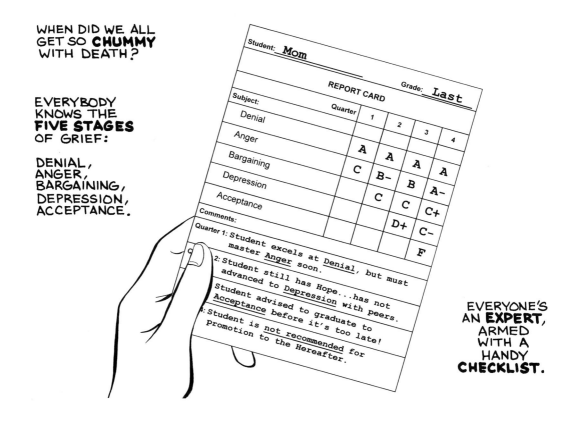

Student: **Mom**

Grade: **Last**

REPORT CARD

Subject: Quarter	1	2	3	4
Denial				
Anger	A	A	A	A
Bargaining	C	B-	A	A
Depression		C	B	A-
Acceptance			C	C+
			D+	C-
				F

Comments:

Quarter 1: Student excels at Denial, but must master Anger soon.

2: Student still has Hope...has not advanced to Depression with peers.

Student advised to graduate to Acceptance before it's too late!

4: Student is not recommended for promotion to the Hereafter.

EVERYONE'S AN **EXPERT,** ARMED WITH A HANDY **CHECKLIST.**

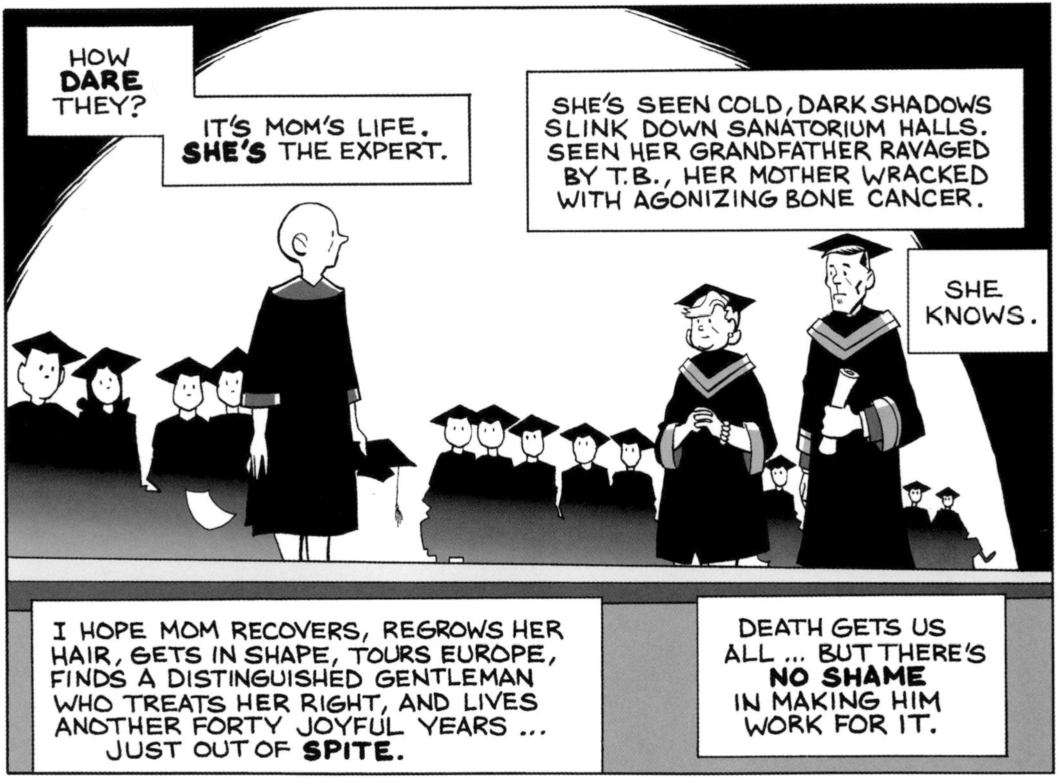
HOW **DARE** THEY?
IT'S MOM'S LIFE. **SHE'S** THE EXPERT.
SHE'S SEEN COLD, DARK SHADOWS SLINK DOWN SANATORIUM HALLS. SEEN HER GRANDFATHER RAVAGED BY T.B., HER MOTHER WRACKED WITH AGONIZING BONE CANCER.
SHE KNOWS.
I HOPE MOM RECOVERS, REGROWS HER HAIR, GETS IN SHAPE, TOURS EUROPE, FINDS A DISTINGUISHED GENTLEMAN WHO TREATS HER RIGHT, AND LIVES ANOTHER FORTY JOYFUL YEARS ... JUST OUT OF **SPITE**.
DEATH GETS US ALL ... BUT THERE'S **NO SHAME** IN MAKING HIM WORK FOR IT.

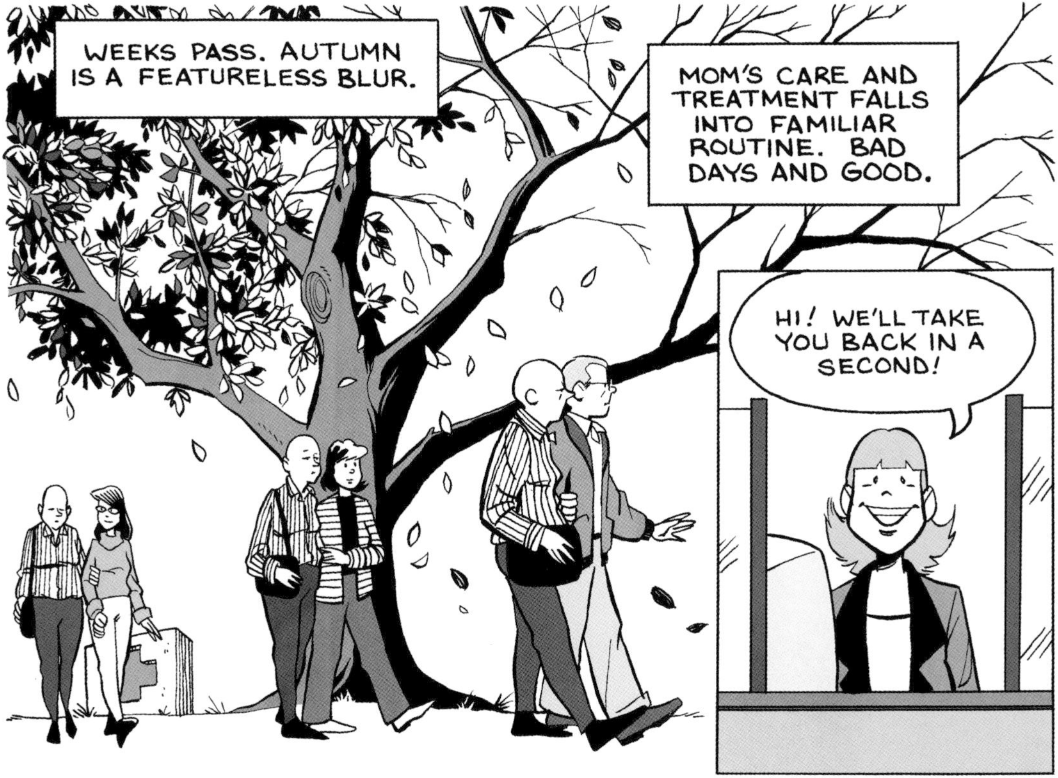
WEEKS PASS. AUTUMN IS A FEATURELESS BLUR.
MOM'S CARE AND TREATMENT FALLS INTO FAMILIAR ROUTINE. BAD DAYS AND GOOD.
HI! WE'LL TAKE YOU BACK IN A SECOND!

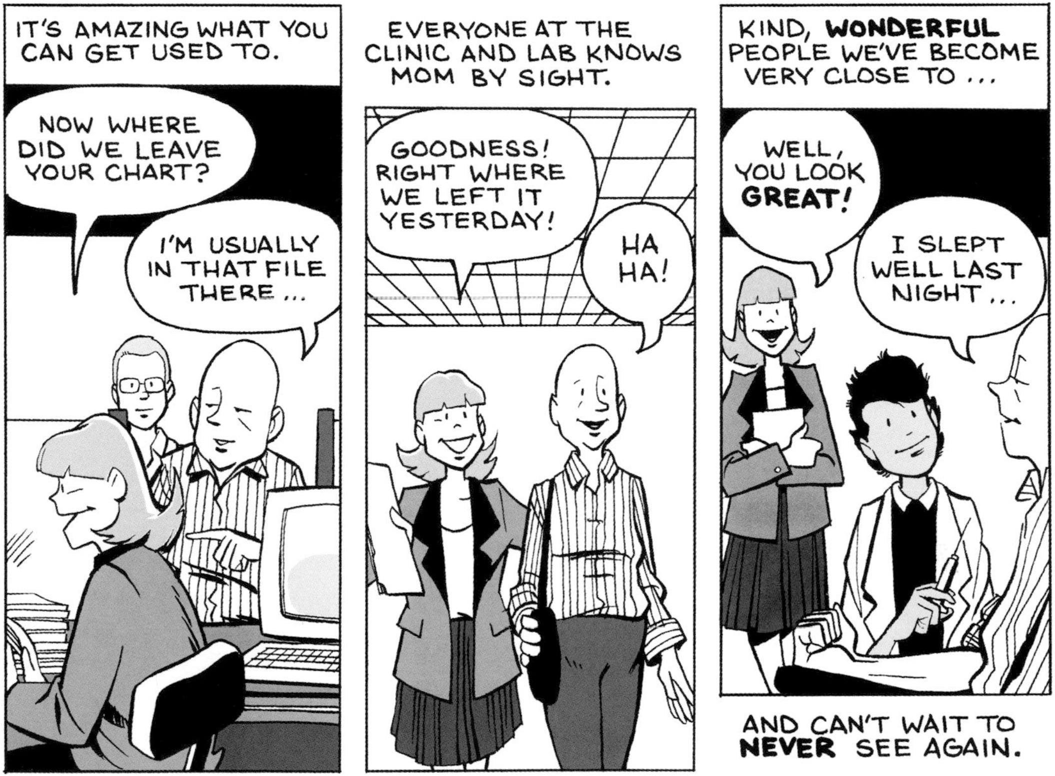
IT'S AMAZING WHAT YOU CAN GET USED TO.
NOW WHERE DID WE LEAVE YOUR CHART?
I'M USUALLY IN THAT FILE THERE ...
EVERYONE AT THE CLINIC AND LAB KNOWS MOM BY SIGHT.
GOODNESS! RIGHT WHERE WE LEFT IT YESTERDAY!
HA HA!
KIND, **WONDERFUL** PEOPLE WE'VE BECOME VERY CLOSE TO ...
WELL, YOU LOOK **GREAT**!
I SLEPT WELL LAST NIGHT ...
AND CAN'T WAIT TO **NEVER** SEE AGAIN.

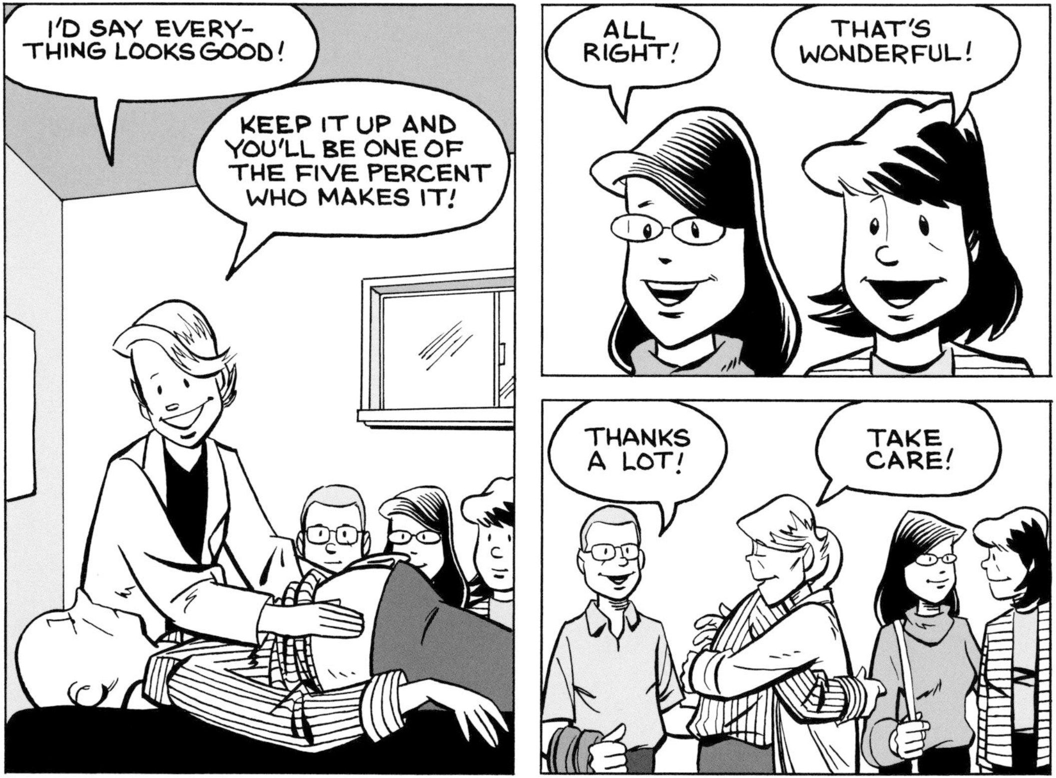
I'D SAY EVERY-THING LOOKS GOOD!
KEEP IT UP AND YOU'LL BE ONE OF THE FIVE PERCENT WHO MAKES IT!
ALL RIGHT!
THAT'S WONDERFUL!
THANKS A LOT!
TAKE CARE!

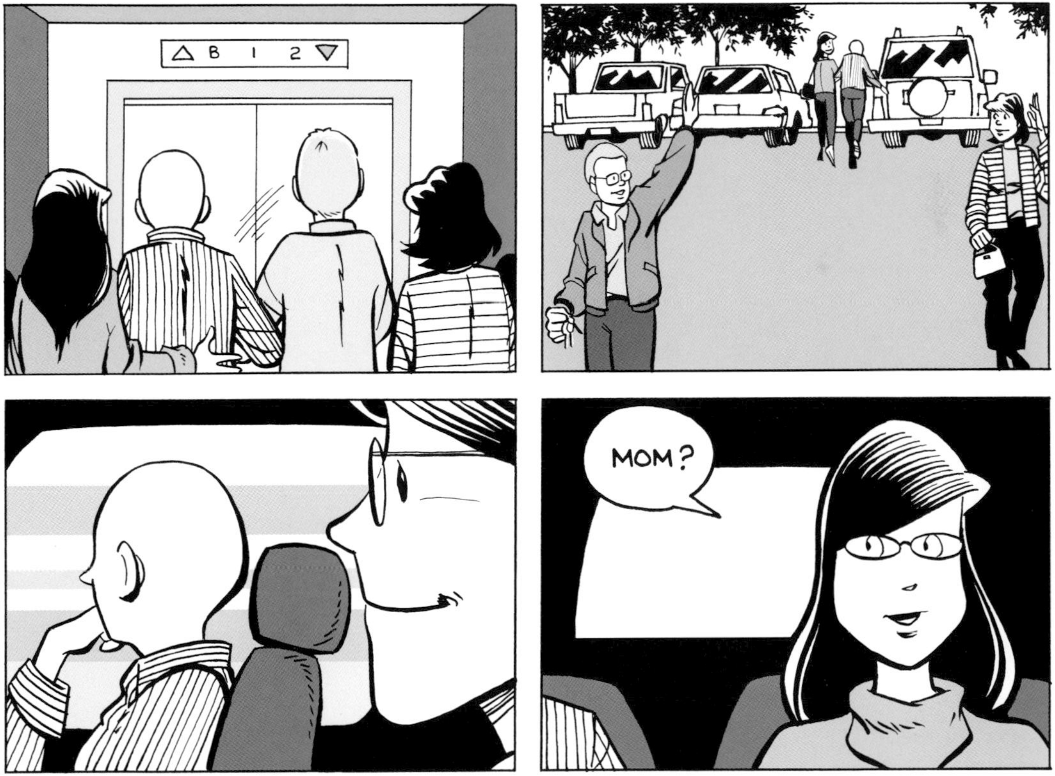
B 1 2
MOM?

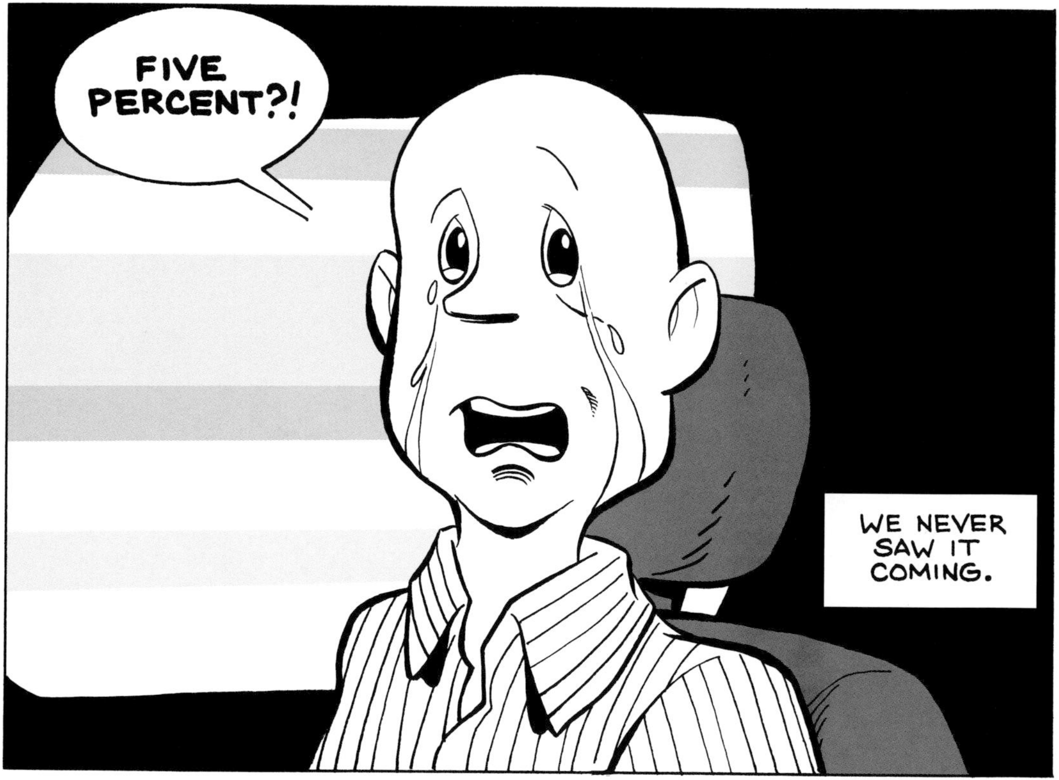
FIVE PERCENT?!
WE NEVER SAW IT COMING.

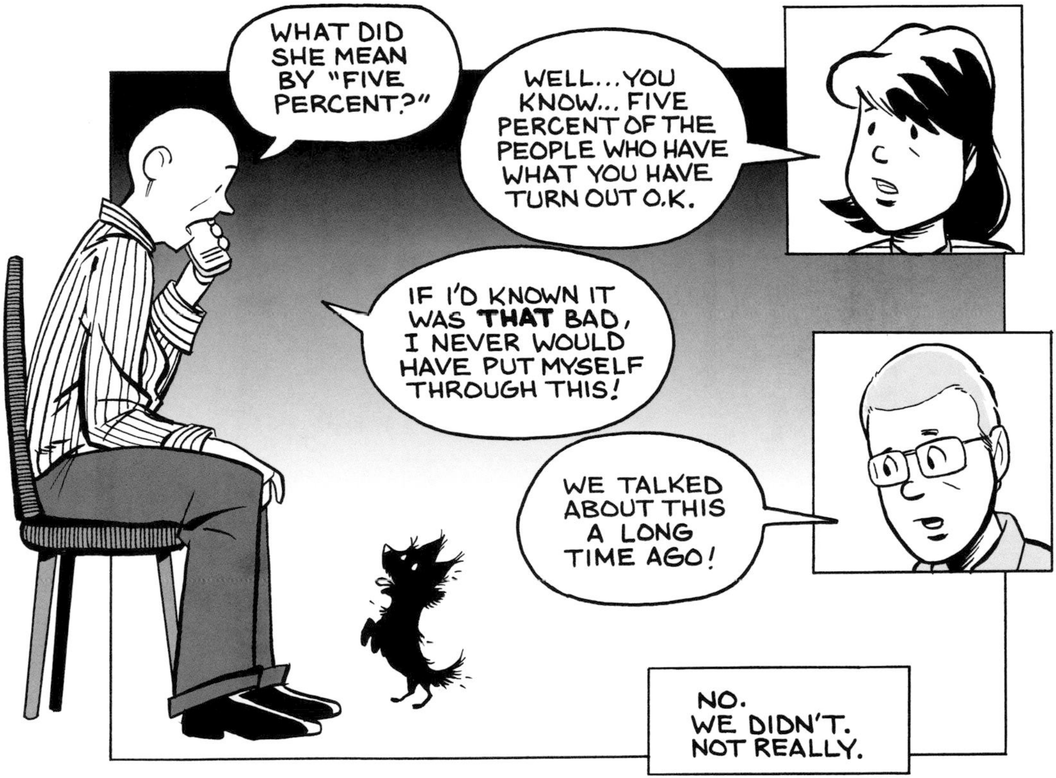

WHAT DID SHE MEAN BY "FIVE PERCENT?"
WELL... YOU KNOW... FIVE PERCENT OF THE PEOPLE WHO HAVE WHAT YOU HAVE TURN OUT O.K.
IF I'D KNOWN IT WAS **THAT** BAD, I NEVER WOULD HAVE PUT MYSELF THROUGH THIS!
WE TALKED ABOUT THIS A LONG TIME AGO!
NO. WE DIDN'T. NOT REALLY.

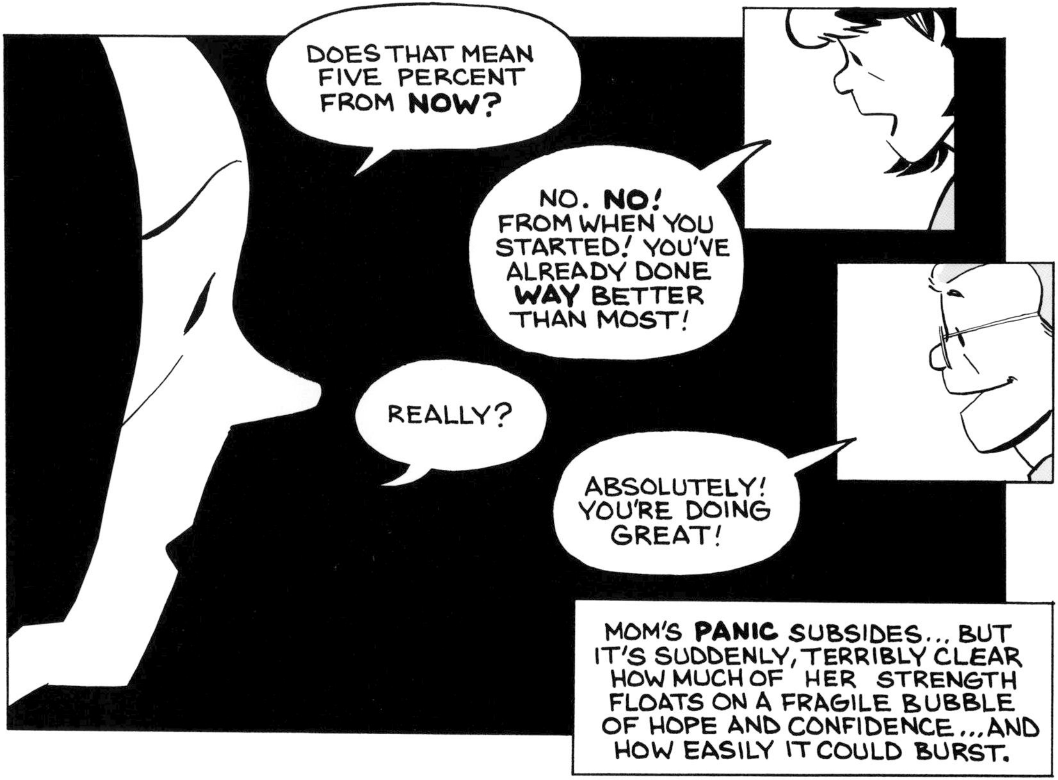
DOES THAT MEAN FIVE PERCENT FROM **NOW?**
NO. **NO!** FROM WHEN YOU STARTED! YOU'VE ALREADY DONE **WAY** BETTER THAN MOST!
REALLY?
ABSOLUTELY! YOU'RE DOING GREAT!
MOM'S **PANIC** SUBSIDES... BUT IT'S SUDDENLY, TERRIBLY CLEAR HOW MUCH OF HER STRENGTH FLOATS ON A FRAGILE BUBBLE OF HOPE AND CONFIDENCE... AND HOW EASILY IT COULD BURST.

WAITING FOR MY WIFE TO GET THE MINIVAN

THERE ARE MOMENTS THAT, EVEN WHILE YOU'RE BUSY LIVING THEM, YOU KNOW YOU'LL REMEMBER FOREVER.

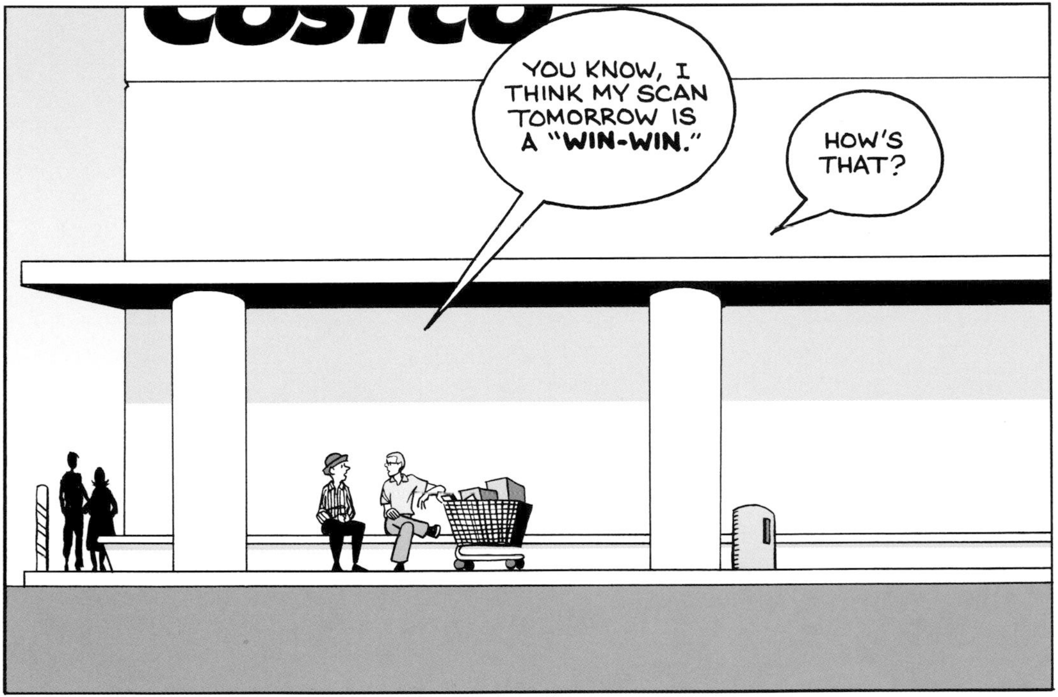
YOU KNOW, I THINK MY SCAN TOMORROW IS A "WIN-WIN."
HOW'S THAT?

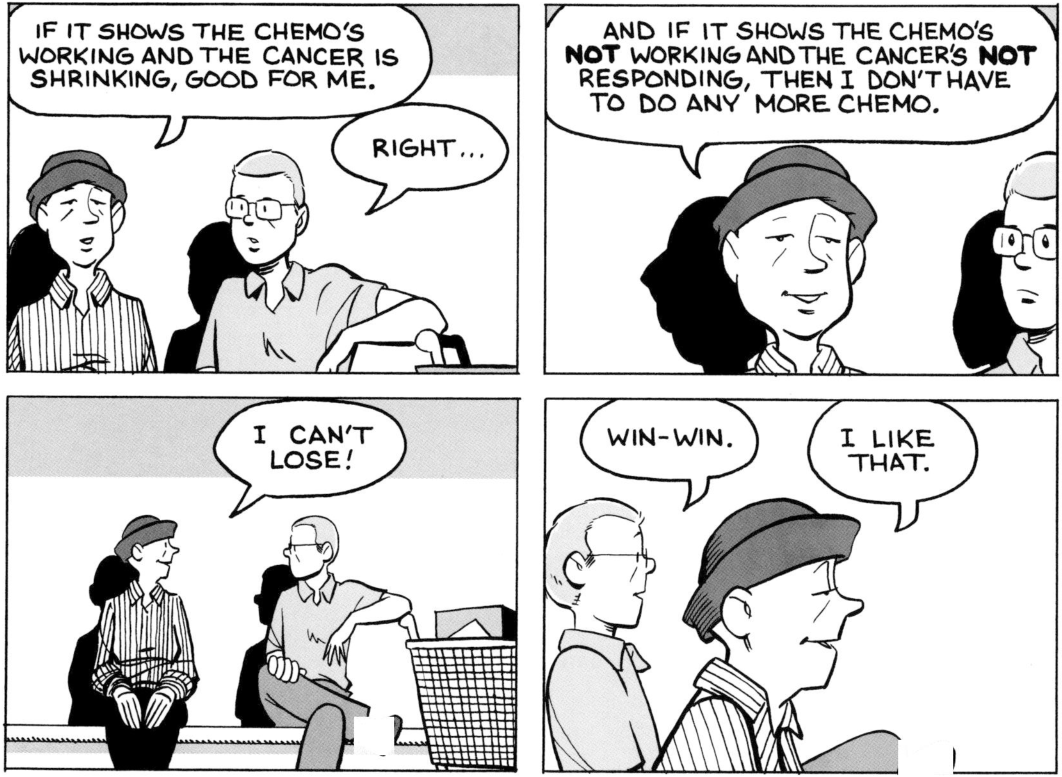
IF IT SHOWS THE CHEMO'S WORKING AND THE CANCER IS SHRINKING, GOOD FOR ME.
RIGHT...
AND IF IT SHOWS THE CHEMO'S NOT WORKING AND THE CANCER'S NOT RESPONDING, THEN I DON'T HAVE TO DO ANY MORE CHEMO.
I CAN'T LOSE!
WIN-WIN.
I LIKE THAT.

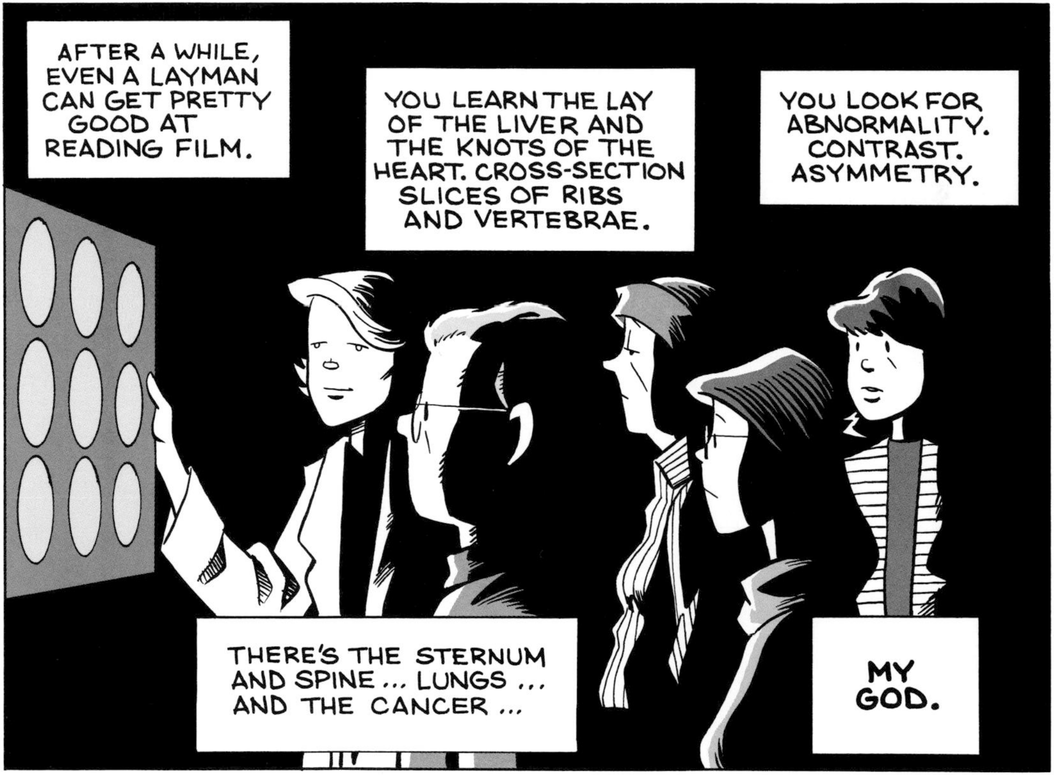
AFTER A WHILE, EVEN A LAYMAN CAN GET PRETTY GOOD AT READING FILM.
YOU LEARN THE LAY OF THE LIVER AND THE KNOTS OF THE HEART. CROSS-SECTION SLICES OF RIBS AND VERTEBRAE.
YOU LOOK FOR ABNORMALITY. CONTRAST. ASYMMETRY.
THERE'S THE STERNUM AND SPINE ... LUNGS ... AND THE CANCER ...
MY GOD.

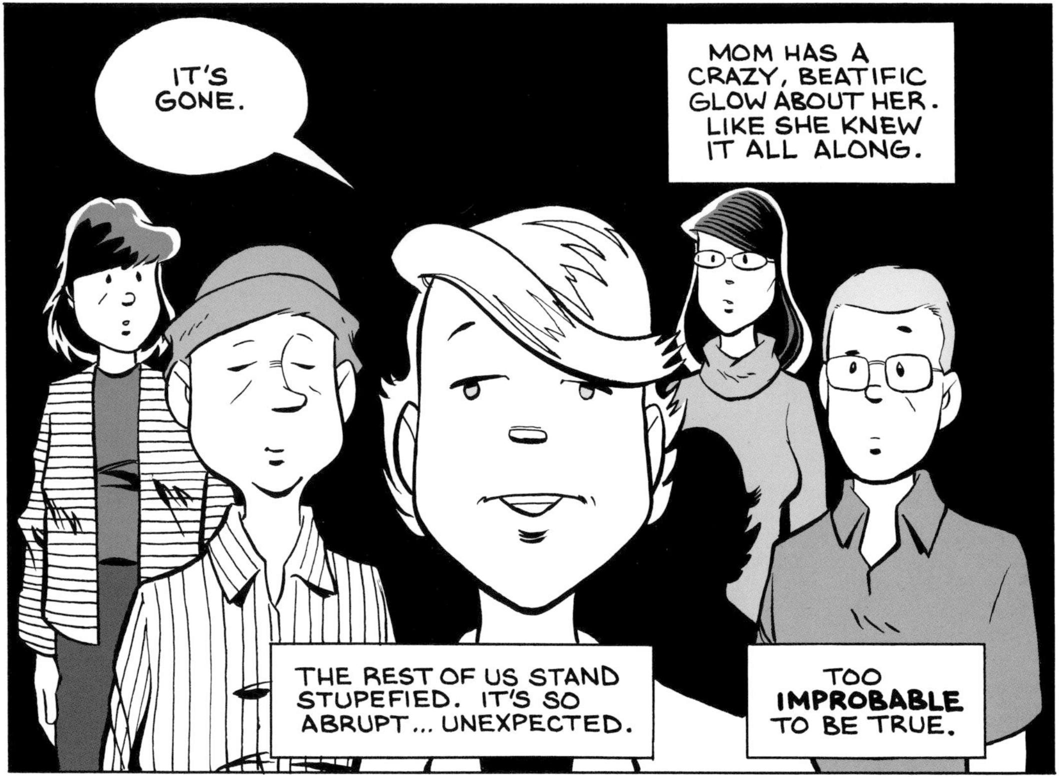
IT'S GONE.
MOM HAS A CRAZY, BEATIFIC GLOW ABOUT HER. LIKE SHE KNEW IT ALL ALONG.
THE REST OF US STAND STUPEFIED. IT'S SO ABRUPT... UNEXPECTED.
TOO **IMPROBABLE** TO BE TRUE.

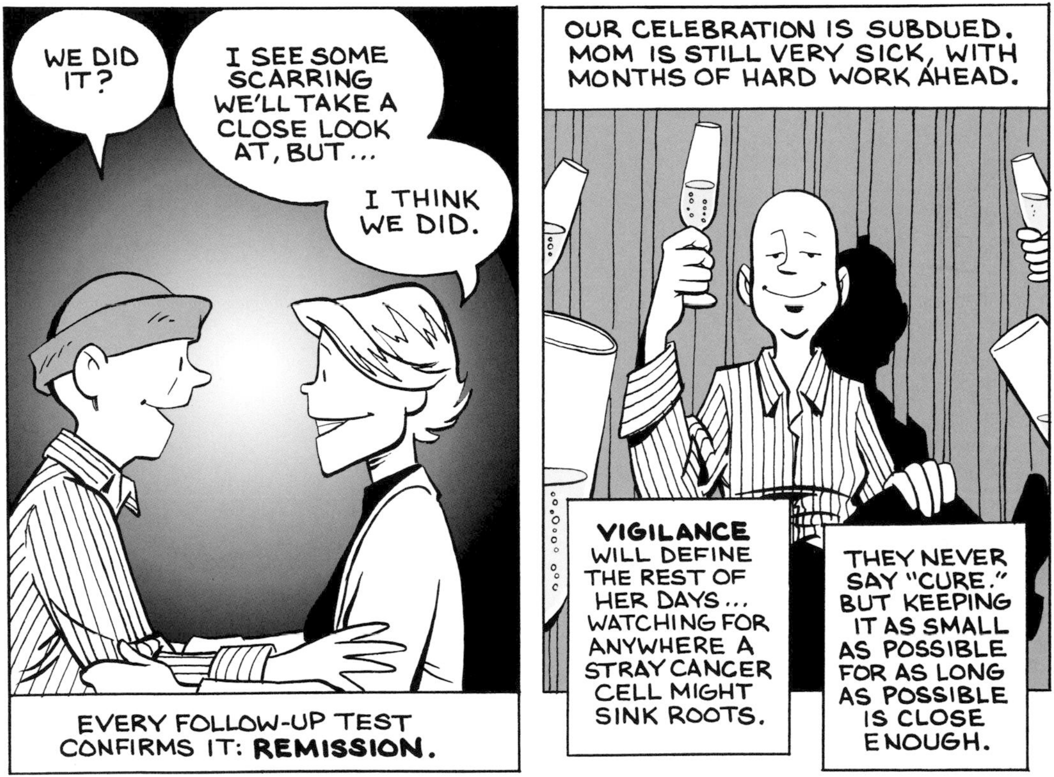
WE DID IT?
I SEE SOME SCARRING WE'LL TAKE A CLOSE LOOK AT, BUT...
I THINK WE DID.
EVERY FOLLOW-UP TEST CONFIRMS IT: **REMISSION**.
OUR CELEBRATION IS SUBDUED. MOM IS STILL VERY SICK, WITH MONTHS OF HARD WORK AHEAD.
VIGILANCE WILL DEFINE THE REST OF HER DAYS... WATCHING FOR ANYWHERE A STRAY CANCER CELL MIGHT SINK ROOTS.
THEY NEVER SAY "CURE." BUT KEEPING IT AS SMALL AS POSSIBLE FOR AS LONG AS POSSIBLE IS CLOSE ENOUGH.

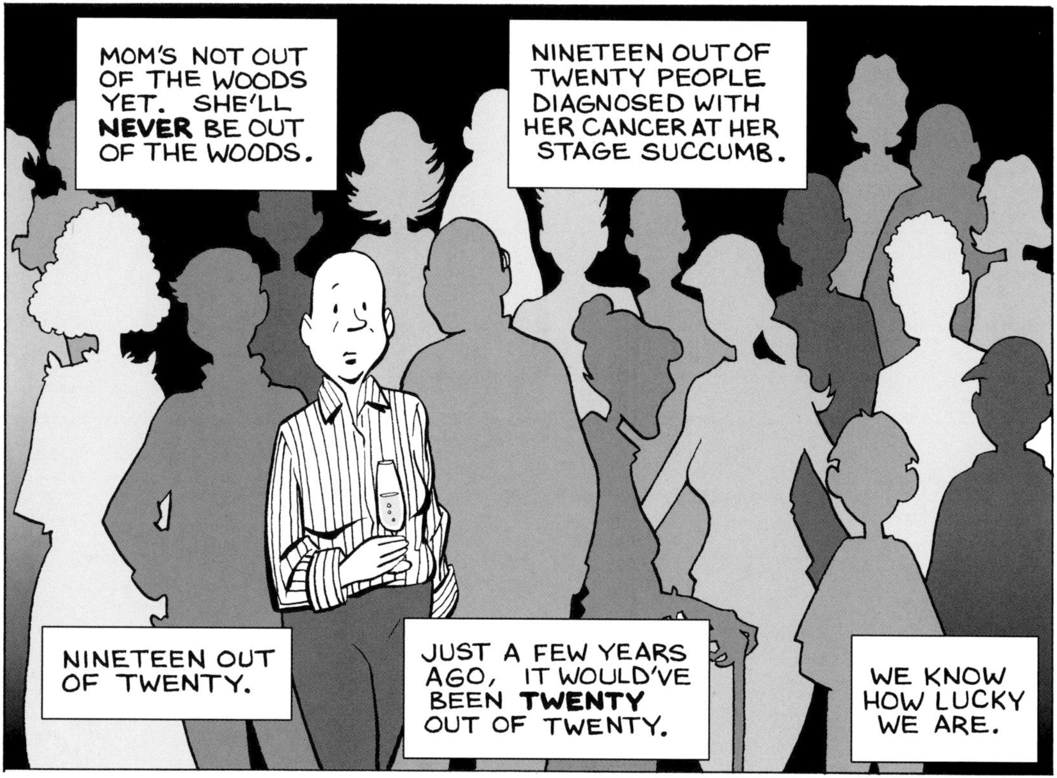
MOM'S NOT OUT OF THE WOODS YET. SHE'LL **NEVER** BE OUT OF THE WOODS.
NINETEEN OUT OF TWENTY PEOPLE DIAGNOSED WITH HER CANCER AT HER STAGE SUCCUMB.
NINETEEN OUT OF TWENTY.
JUST A FEW YEARS AGO, IT WOULD'VE BEEN **TWENTY** OUT OF TWENTY.
WE KNOW HOW LUCKY WE ARE.

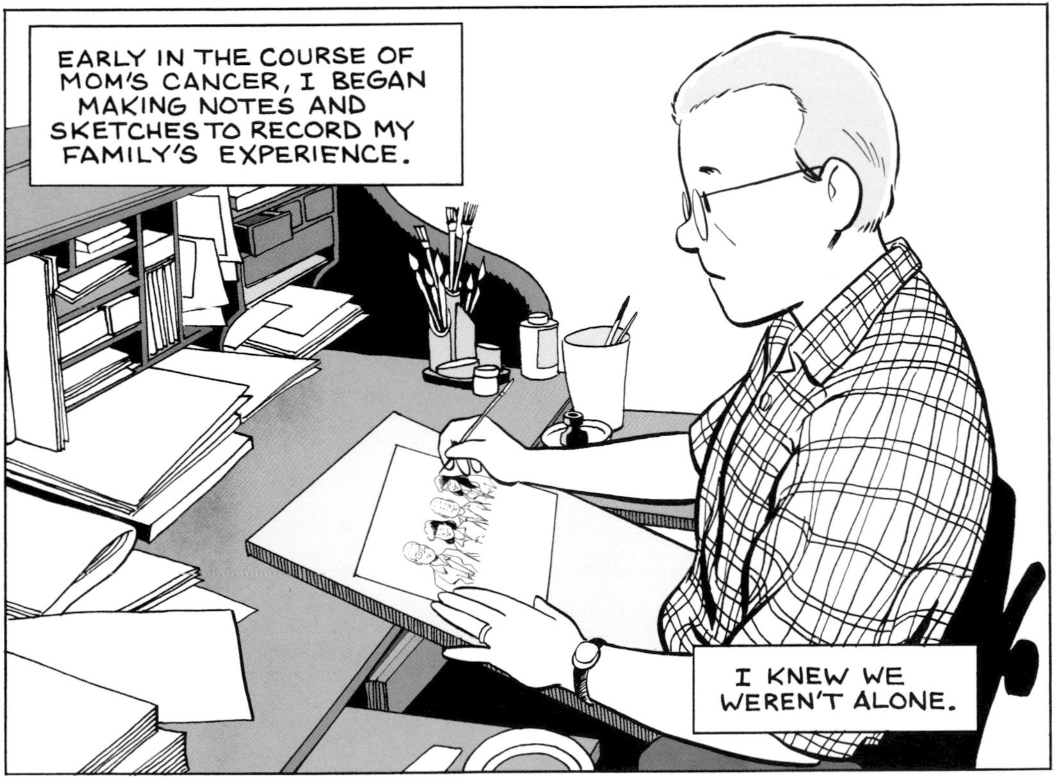
EARLY IN THE COURSE OF MOM'S CANCER, I BEGAN MAKING NOTES AND SKETCHES TO RECORD MY FAMILY'S EXPERIENCE.
I KNEW WE WEREN'T ALONE.

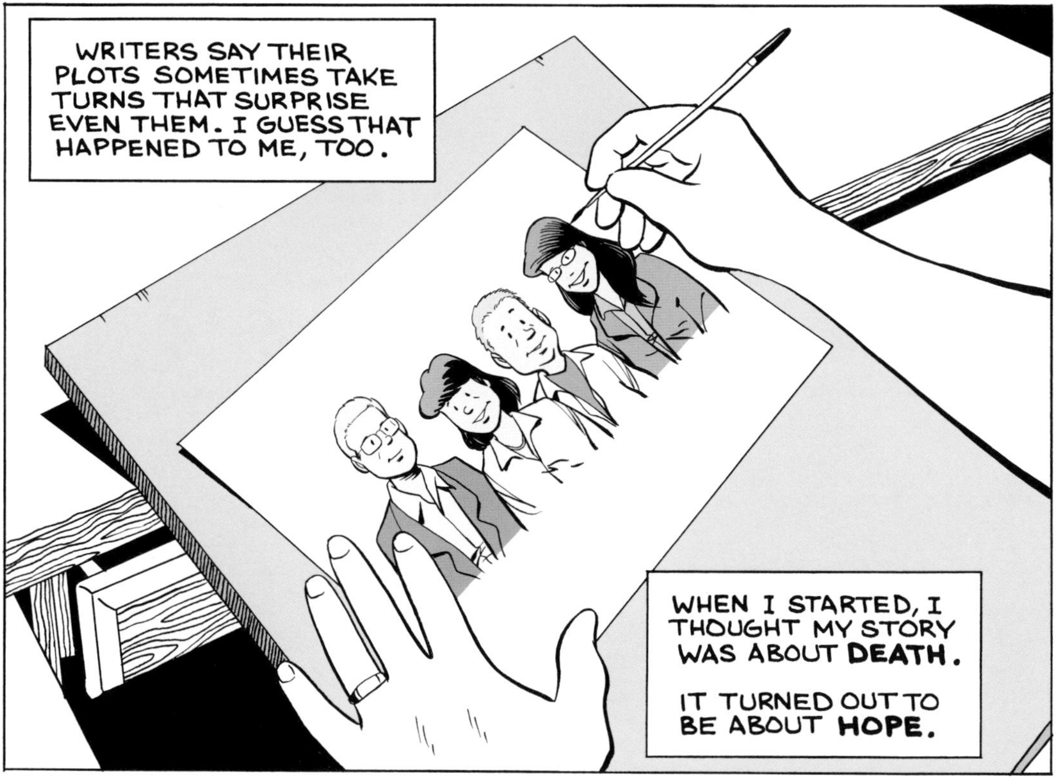
WRITERS SAY THEIR PLOTS SOMETIMES TAKE TURNS THAT SURPRISE EVEN THEM. I GUESS THAT HAPPENED TO ME, TOO.
WHEN I STARTED, I THOUGHT MY STORY WAS ABOUT **DEATH**.
IT TURNED OUT TO BE ABOUT **HOPE**.

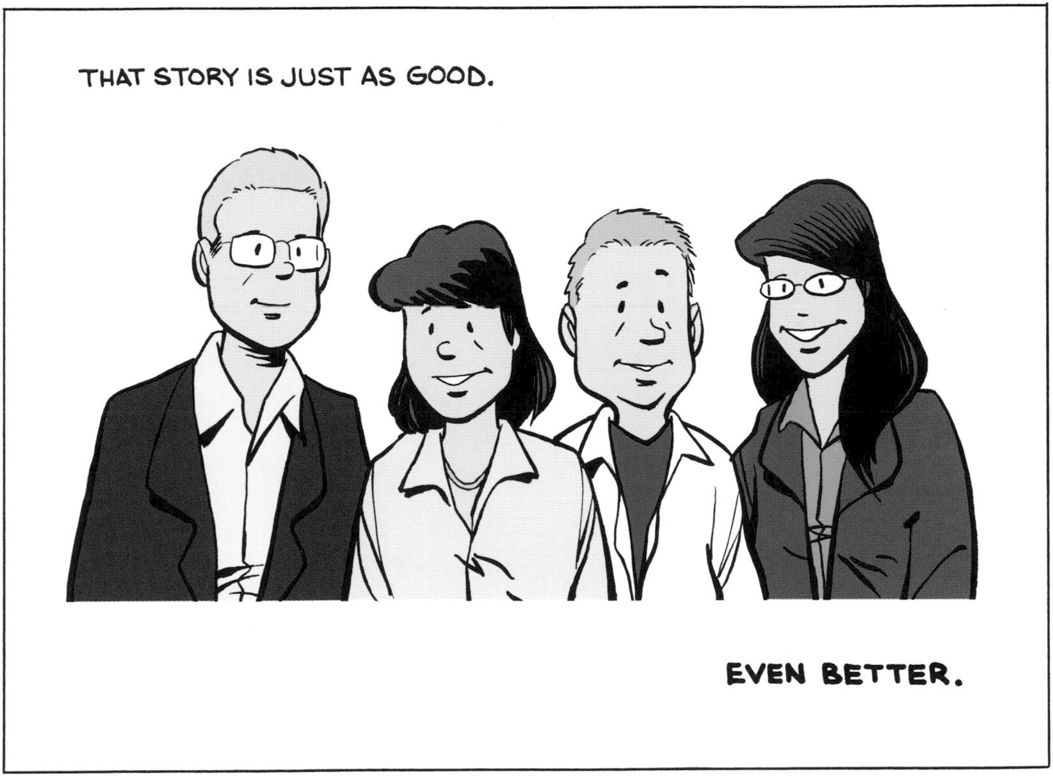
THAT STORY IS JUST AS GOOD.
EVEN BETTER.

AN EPILOGUE

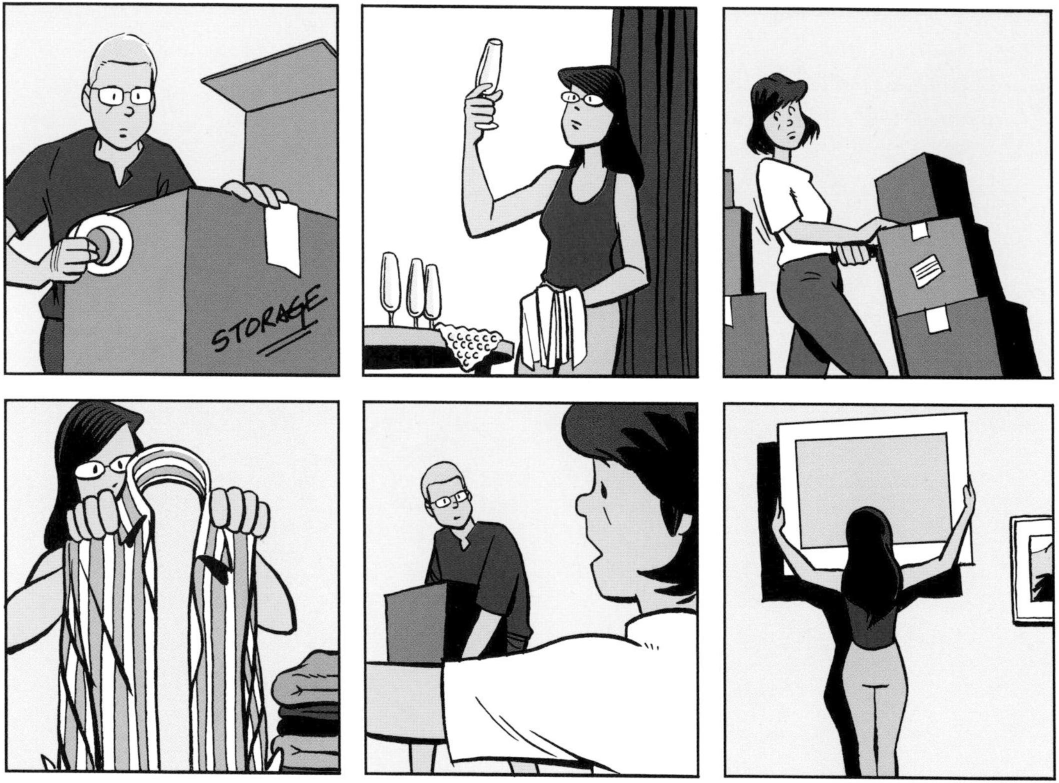
STORAGE

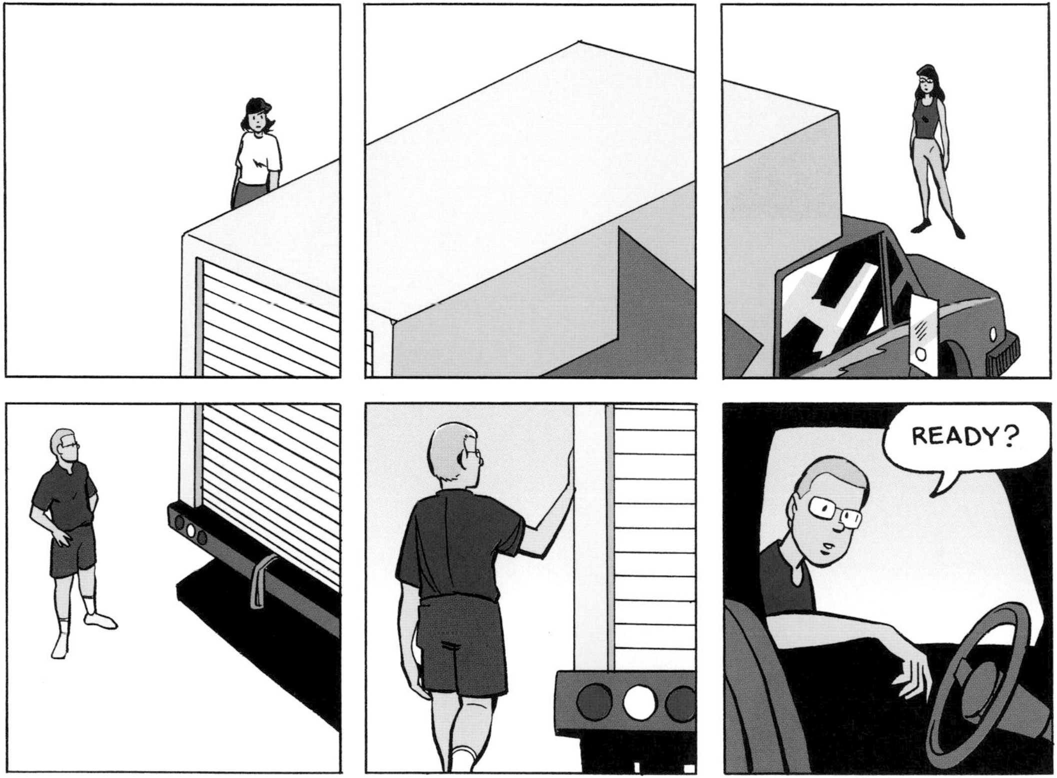
READY?

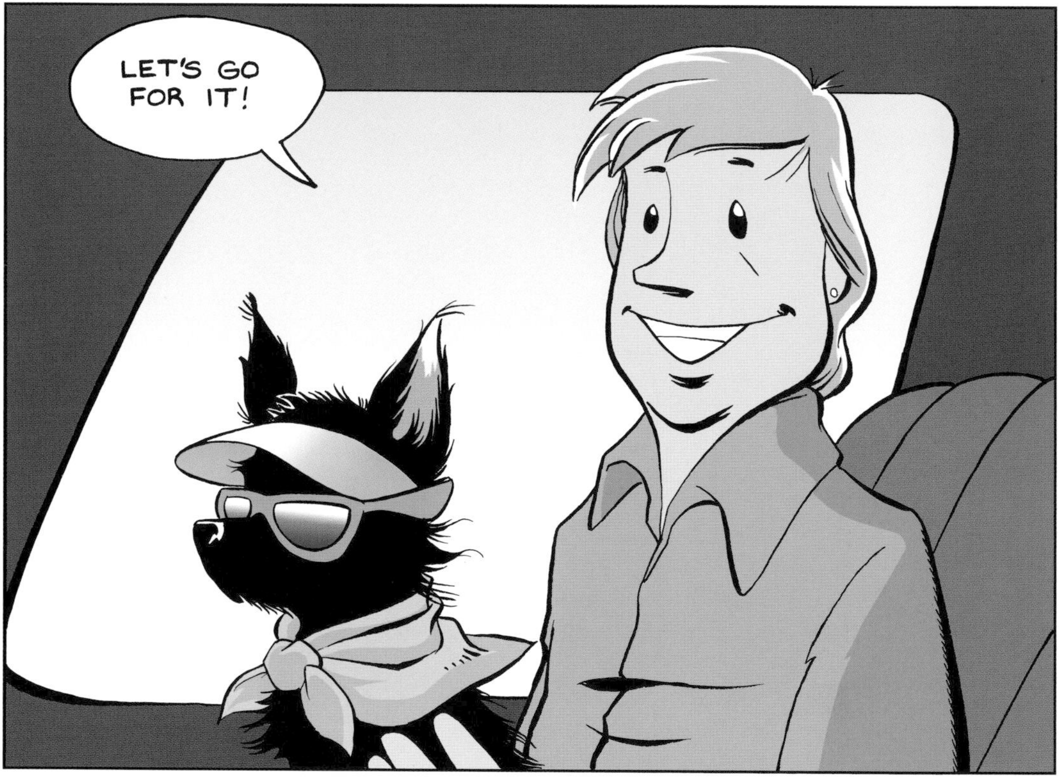
LET'S GO FOR IT!

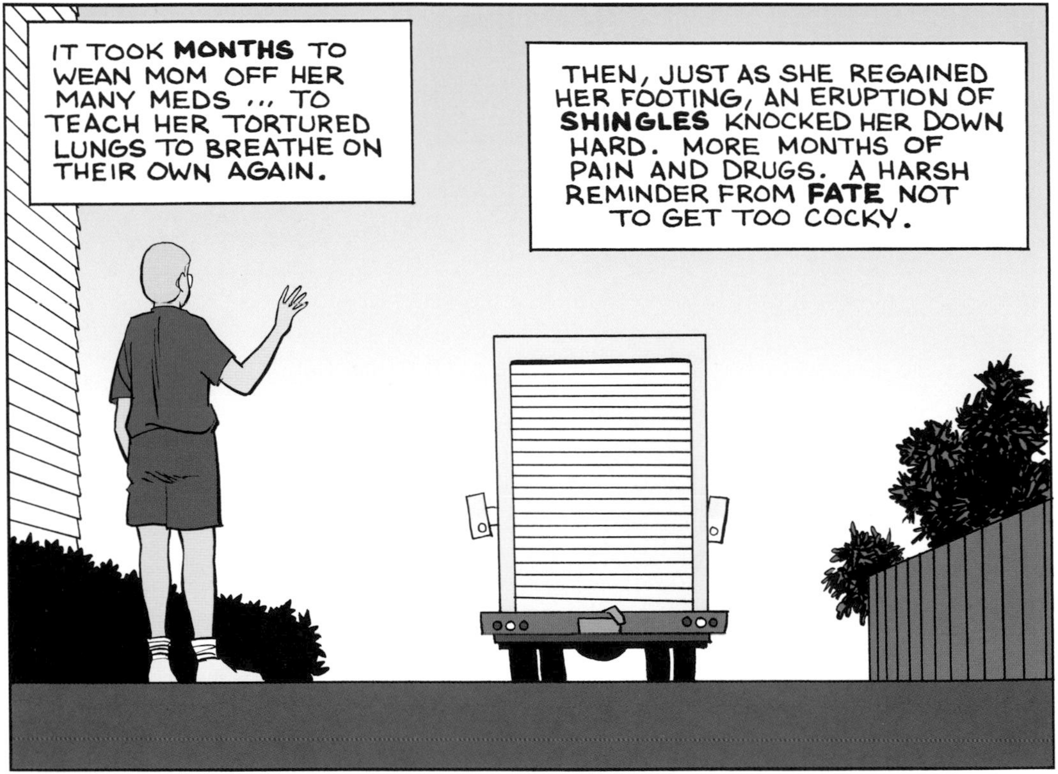
IT TOOK MONTHS TO WEAN MOM OFF HER MANY MEDS ... TO TEACH HER TORTURED LUNGS TO BREATHE ON THEIR OWN AGAIN.
THEN, JUST AS SHE REGAINED HER FOOTING, AN ERUPTION OF SHINGLES KNOCKED HER DOWN HARD. MORE MONTHS OF PAIN AND DRUGS. A HARSH REMINDER FROM FATE NOT TO GET TOO COCKY.

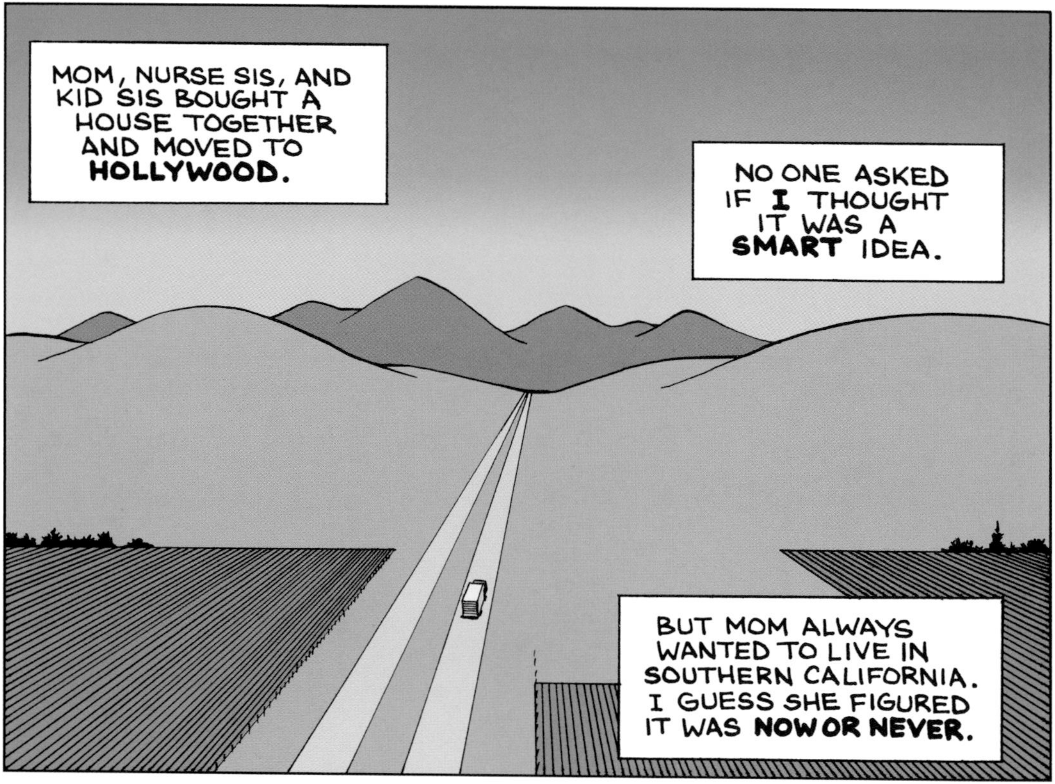
MOM, NURSE SIS, AND KID SIS BOUGHT A HOUSE TOGETHER AND MOVED TO **HOLLYWOOD.**
NO ONE ASKED IF **I** THOUGHT IT WAS A **SMART** IDEA.
BUT MOM ALWAYS WANTED TO LIVE IN SOUTHERN CALIFORNIA. I GUESS SHE FIGURED IT WAS **NOW OR NEVER.**

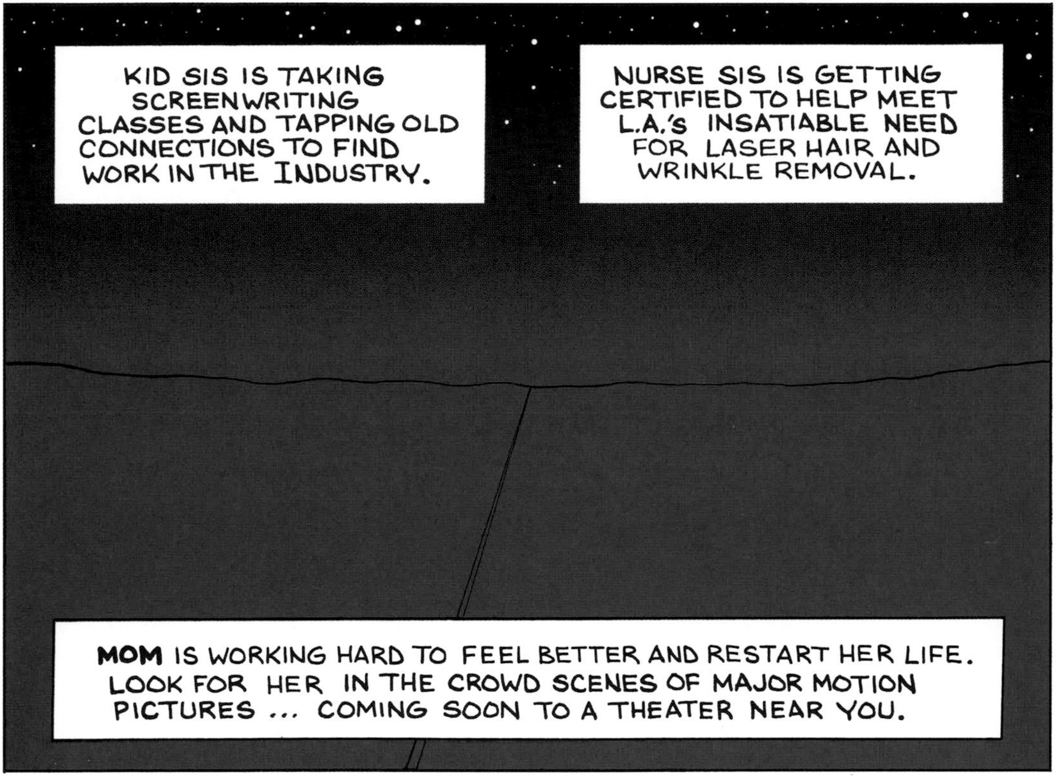
KID SIS IS TAKING SCREENWRITING CLASSES AND TAPPING OLD CONNECTIONS TO FIND WORK IN THE INDUSTRY.
NURSE SIS IS GETTING CERTIFIED TO HELP MEET L.A.'s INSATIABLE NEED FOR LASER HAIR AND WRINKLE REMOVAL.
MOM IS WORKING HARD TO FEEL BETTER AND RESTART HER LIFE. LOOK FOR HER IN THE CROWD SCENES OF MAJOR MOTION PICTURES ... COMING SOON TO A THEATER NEAR YOU.

AFTERWORD

When I found out about *Mom's Cancer* my first thought was, "Oh no! I wish it could be about something great I've done with my life." To have my soft underbelly exposed was difficult. Then I realized I was still anonymous—just "Mom" unless I chose to tell someone. My pride in Brian's work and fascination with the depth of the story made the telling worthwhile. He also made me look a lot better than I felt!

People thought we were crazy when we moved to southern California. But it was important for me to take charge of what was left of my life and do something that could actually add to its quality. I wanted to be somewhere I felt vibrant and alive, with sunshine, great food, cultural events, and good friends planning fun things to do. I never felt I was leaving the old hometown or all of my dear friends and family for good. I was just expanding. We found a beautiful home in a quiet, caring, established neighborhood where people wave and call each other by name. It feels more like home than home did.

It's too soon to know what I've learned from all this. I know the most important person for me to take care of now is me, so that I will be around to help others later. Of all the things I've done, I am least proud of smoking—and now that's what I'm getting recognized for. It's hard to separate that in my mind and remember that *Mom's Cancer* is about the process and, most important, the family. What got me through treatment was an almost blind determination that I could win out over a cigarette. It was not going to take me down! I have good days and bad days, and sometimes it's hard to tell the difference. But I'm learning not to expect so much of myself. I'm learning to be more grateful for the body parts that do decide to work on any given day. And I'm still looking for Mr. Right.

The fatigue I experienced was the worst of my life. I got so bone-tired I didn't know how many more windmills I could fight. Day after day, it took all I had to raise my hand or shift position. The biggest surprise for me was that I didn't feel like myself as soon as treatment stopped. Remission doesn't mean you're going to be who you were. During the process of chemotherapy and radiation, the doctors take a lot of the good cells, too.

Asking for help is hard but necessary. Anyone confronting a life-altering health issue should delegate as much as possible from the very beginning. I just knew I could wash my own laundry, find something to eat, and keep doing it all. But suddenly I couldn't even count out my meds for the day, balance a checkbook, or take a phone message. I hadn't realized how strong the drugs were, how fast they'd built up in my system, and how unlike myself I'd become. How dense the fog really was (and still is). I thought I was doing fine. Instead, I leaned way too hard on my two closest caregivers, my daughters. They've been right beside me all along, so willing to lend a hand, and I let them. Worse, I expected them to. It seems that it took all of us to keep me alive. Now, hopefully, all of us can have a great new beginning to our own dreams and goals.

Technology is moving so quickly and lives being saved so miraculously that doctors can't keep up. More and more people are living, but with less and less quality of life. We're limping around in foreign, broken bodies, filled with "chemo brains" and radiation, wondering where our selves went and if we'll ever come back. We need cancer treatment programs that include detoxing, physical and occupational therapy, exercise classes, pampering, and understanding. We need honest information on how to take care of ourselves when fingernails sheer off until they bleed. What to do when our hands and feet tingle until we want to cut them off. What to do when pain rips through our brains like a tornado. We need the truth.

Cherish rest, laughter, friends, and prayers. Trust in yourself and make a peace treaty with your Higher Power. Have a Hero to never let go of and help you through the terrifying nights. Take frequent baths to get rid of the scent of toxins. Watch a lot of comedies. Keep your mind and hands busy. Then just breathe for as long as you can, knowing that others are helping to hold you up.

"Mom"
Hollywood, California
2005

FOR MORE INFORMATION

The following organizations and websites are among many established to provide information, advocacy, and support for those fighting lung cancer and related diseases.

American Cancer Society, 800-ACS-2345, www.cancer.org
American Lung Association, 800-LUNGUSA, www.lungusa.org
Association of Cancer Online Resources, www.acor.org
CancerCare.org, 800-813-HOPE, www.cancercare.org
Cancer.net, www.cancer.net
ClinicalTrials.gov (U.S. National Institutes of Health and the National Library of Medicine), www.clinicaltrials.gov
Lung Cancer Alliance, www.lungcanceralliance.org
LungCancer.org, 877-646-LUNG, www.lungcancer.org
Lung Cancer Support Community, www.lchelp.com
National Cancer Institute, www.cancer.gov
National Lung Cancer Partnership, www.nationallungcancerpartnership.org
OncoLink, www.oncolink.org